The
Teenage Human Bod
OPERATOR'S MANUAL

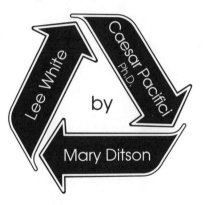

by

Lee White

Caesar Pacifici Ph.D.

Mary Ditson

Graphic Design: Ric Harbin

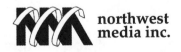

northwest media inc.

Support for this program was provided to Northwest Media, Inc. through a grant from the National Institute of Child Health and Human Development, Small Business Innovation Research Project #2 R44 HD30649-02. The content of this program, including mention of trade names and commercial products, is not intended to reflect the views, policies, or endorsement of the United States Government.

Northwest Media, Inc.
326 West 12th Avenue
Eugene, OR 97401

Telephone: 541-343-6636
FAX: 541-343-0177

e-mail: nwm@northwestmedia.com
web page: http://www.northwestmedia.com

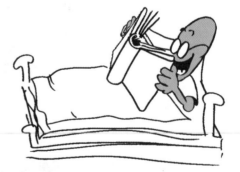

ISBN 1-892194-01-5 • Library of Congress Catalog Number: 98-86221

Special thanks to: **Robert Nickel, M.D.**
Mollie Davis, Student, South Eugene High School
Martha Debroeker, R.N., Lane County Public Health Services
Susan Fries, R.N.-C., F.N.P., South Eugene School-Based Health Center
Marilyn Stevens, R.N., Eugene School District Health Services
Sexual Assault Support Services, Eugene, Oregon

About the Artist

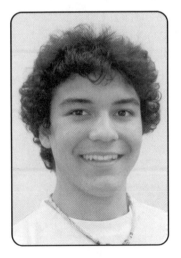

Mike Novotny showed a passion for drawing before he could walk or talk. This passion fueled the talent with which Mike won many drawing contests. In school, Mike's drive to draw caused many of his teachers to say, "Are you paying attention?" But finally, in the fifth grade, Mike had a teacher who appreciated his ability. She encouraged him to complete his assignments in the form of Mind Maps. And when she gave seminars for other teachers, she put Mike in front with markers and easel, making him a visual "interpreter," showing concepts with pictures.

Mike, now 18, is thinking of pursuing art as a career. He would like to create drawings for T-shirts, skateboards and surfboards. This is his first published work and he says, "It's been cool. It will be fun to see a whole book of my drawings." We know you'll have fun seeing his drawings, too.

To those of you who have a passion, like drawing, Mike's suggestion is just, "Go with the flow."

Our General Disclaimer

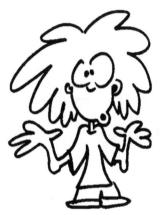

The information published in **The Teenage Human Body Operator's Manual** is offered only for general information and educational purposes. It is not offered as and does not constitute medical advice or medical opinions. Although we intend to keep this information current, we do not promise or guarantee that the information is correct, complete or up-to-date. You should not act or rely upon the information in this publication without seeking the advice of an expert or a doctor.

Table of Contents

Introduction

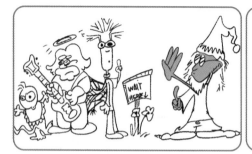 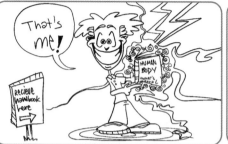 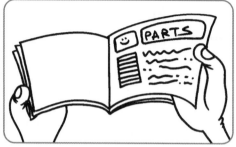

Congratulations!

You own a world-class vehicle — the teenage human body. Countless years of super-engineering have gone into its design.

This Manual

To ensure that you will enjoy many years of trouble-free operation, we have developed this **Operator's Manual**. It is full of valuable information on how to maintain your body. Please read it carefully. Keep it in a safe place for future reference.

Parts

There are eleven parts in this manual. Each part begins with a list of topics, so that you can tell at a glance if it contains the information you want.

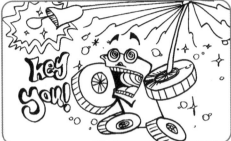

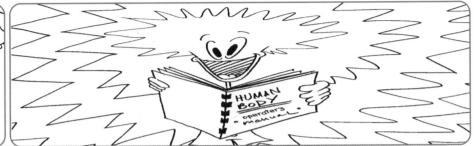

There are many safety warnings in this manual.

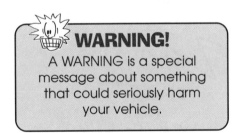

WARNING!

A WARNING is a special message about something that could seriously harm your vehicle.

Using This Manual

A quick way of locating the information you need is to look up related words in the **Index** (in the back), which will send you to specific pages.

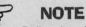 **NOTE**

Following the recommendations in this manual may enhance the performance of your body, but do not use it as a substitute for proper medical care.

For any prolonged symptoms or concerns, see a qualified health care provider.

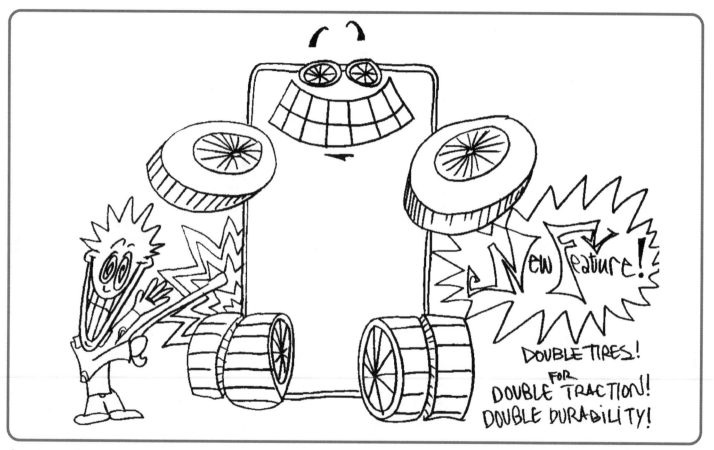

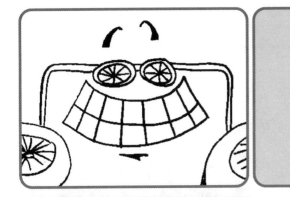

Part 1

Parts and Features

Learn about a few of the standard parts and features of your body.

"You are a system of levers, pumps, and bellows. You are electrical charges and chemical reactions. You are a furnace, filters and a fancy computer with a vast memory bank. You are a finely tuned organism with more living parts than New York City, all operating in harmony. When you think about it, you are pretty incredible."

This quote and information on following diagram are from Linda Allison's **Blood and Guts**, The Yolla Bolly Press, 1976.

Parts and Features

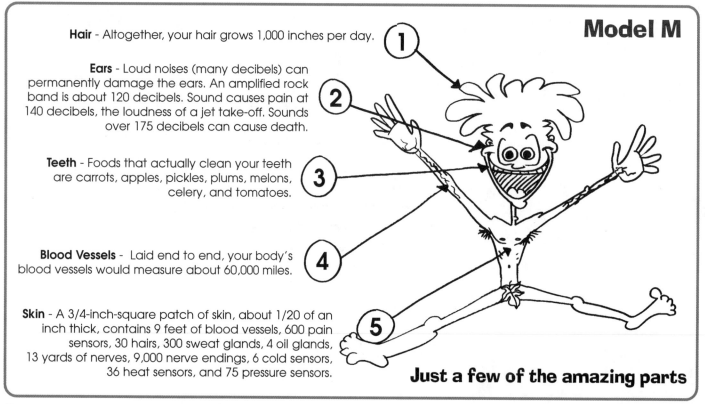

Model M

Hair - Altogether, your hair grows 1,000 inches per day.

Ears - Loud noises (many decibels) can permanently damage the ears. An amplified rock band is about 120 decibels. Sound causes pain at 140 decibels, the loudness of a jet take-off. Sounds over 175 decibels can cause death.

Teeth - Foods that actually clean your teeth are carrots, apples, pickles, plums, melons, celery, and tomatoes.

Blood Vessels - Laid end to end, your body's blood vessels would measure about 60,000 miles.

Skin - A 3/4-inch-square patch of skin, about 1/20 of an inch thick, contains 9 feet of blood vessels, 600 pain sensors, 30 hairs, 300 sweat glands, 4 oil glands, 13 yards of nerves, 9,000 nerve endings, 6 cold sensors, 36 heat sensors, and 75 pressure sensors.

Just a few of the amazing parts

Model F

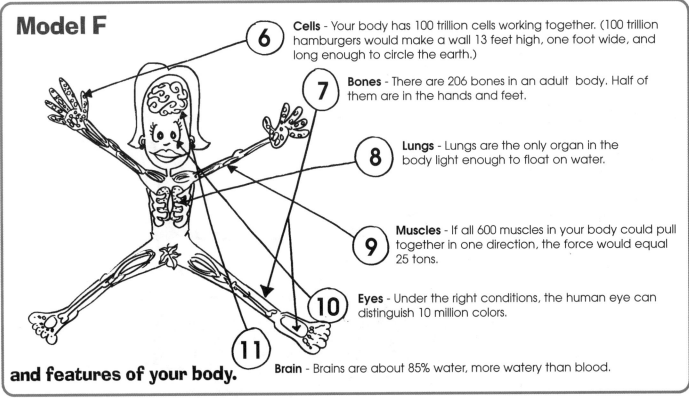

Cells - Your body has 100 trillion cells working together. (100 trillion hamburgers would make a wall 13 feet high, one foot wide, and long enough to circle the earth.)

Bones - There are 206 bones in an adult body. Half of them are in the hands and feet.

Lungs - Lungs are the only organ in the body light enough to float on water.

Muscles - If all 600 muscles in your body could pull together in one direction, the force would equal 25 tons.

Eyes - Under the right conditions, the human eye can distinguish 10 million colors.

Brain - Brains are about 85% water, more watery than blood.

and features of your body.

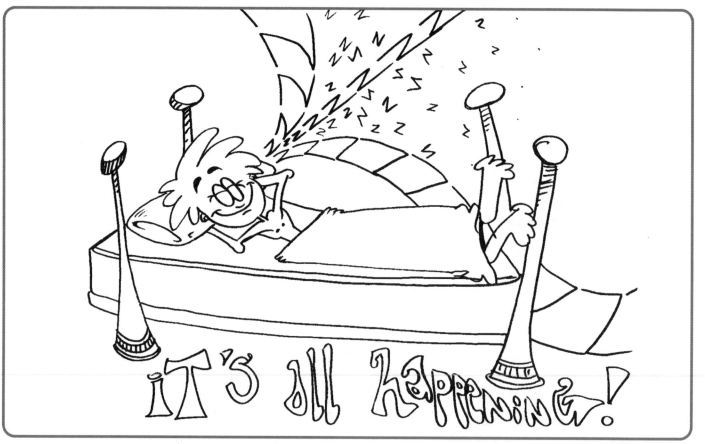

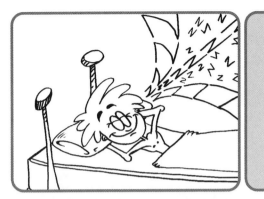

In this part, you'll find information on the operation of the standard systems included in your teenage body.

Automatic Operations

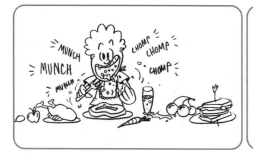

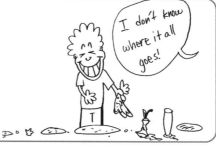

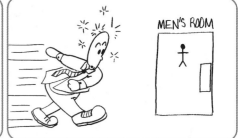

You Don't Even Have to Think About It

Your body is equipped with a significant number of features that operate <u>automatically</u>.

Digestion

Feed your body, and your stomach, intestines, etc. will <u>automatically</u> take care of the job of moving, churning, breaking down and converting food into energy.

Waste Management

At the "tail" end of the digestive process, your body comes with a feature for disposing of its own waste. Generally, you will receive a signal just before this occurs. Place your body in a convenient location as soon as possible.

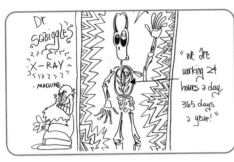

Respiratory & Cardiovascular Systems

Your body needs oxygen to work. Systems that keep the heart beating, the lungs breathing, and vessels moving oxygenated blood to all body parts are in constant <u>automatic</u> operation.

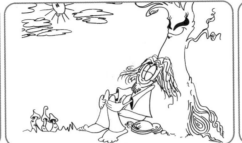

Quiet Mode

When your body is idling (relaxing), your breathing, digestion and heart rate <u>automatically</u> slow down.

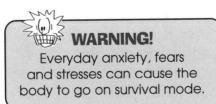

WARNING!
Everyday anxiety, fears and stresses can cause the body to go on survival mode.

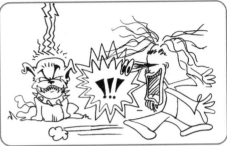

Survival Mode

If your survival is threatened, your biochemical system will <u>automatically</u> shift — breathing and heart rate will speed up and more blood will be sent to the muscles — so you can run, or fight, for your life.

Automatic Operations

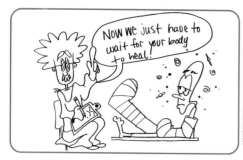

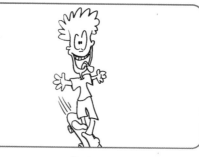

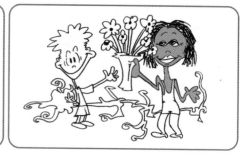

Automatic Healing

One of the most remarkable features of your body is that it will heal <u>automatically</u> from many problems. Skin, blood vessels, bones, and muscles restore themselves after being torn or broken. White blood cells march into infected areas and surround intruding germs.

Automatic Changes

The teen body is programmed for big changes to happen at a genetically determined time. Pubic hair and underarm hair sprout. Boys get facial hair, a low voice, and wet dreams. Girls get their period, more pronounced hips and breasts. Everybody gets sexual feelings.

Automatic Responsibility

As the teen body goes through puberty, the female body produces eggs and the male body produces sperm. Fertilizing an egg with a sperm will <u>automatically</u> start construction of a baby body.

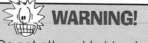

WARNING!

Do not attempt to blend egg and sperm before reading "Sex Brakes" and "Passenger Safety."

14

HOW I GOT TO BE WHERE I AM

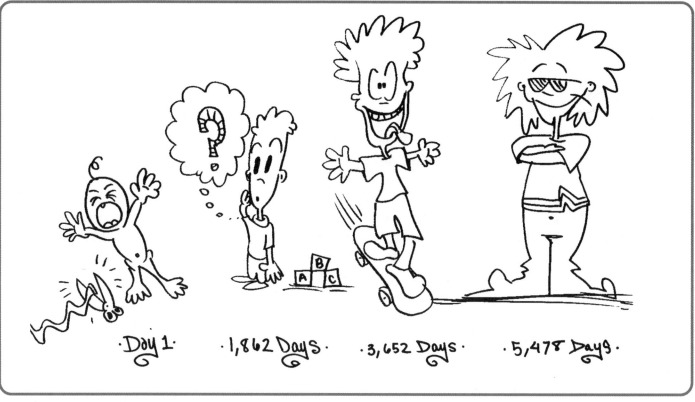

Basic Operations

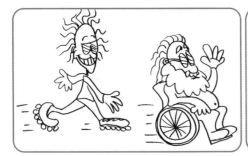

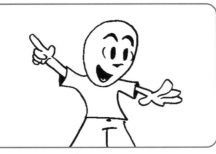

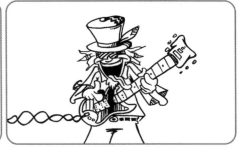

Basic Mobility
Your body has been programmed to learn how to get around and is adapted for a wide range of movement ability.

> 👉 **NOTE**
> Due to excellent original programming, the body can adapt to losing parts or functions.

Basic Language
Your brain is programmed to learn language. The body's language instruments (vocal cords, brain, etc.) can learn to speak any of the world's 200 languages.

Basic Manual Coordination
Using a two-hand system and an opposable thumb feature, your body can perform complex tasks of grasping and manipulating objects.

Operator's Manual

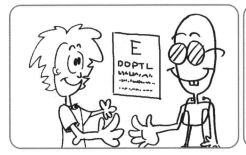

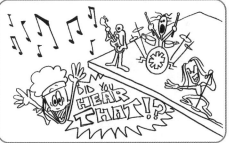

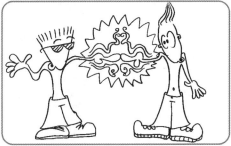

Basic Vision

Your human body has two auto-focus, front-facing eyes, enabling you to see depth (near-far). This allows you to dance, drive, play baseball, etc. Your eyes can also see color in great detail.

Basic Hearing

Your body comes with the ability to hear a wide (frequency) range of sounds and, due to the ear's remarkable construction, to know where the sound is coming from and what it is.

Basic Touch

The skin of your body is sensitive enough to pick up even very subtle differences in temperature and pressure. This sense, like the others, is wired into your brain so that you can understand and use information.

High Performance Operations

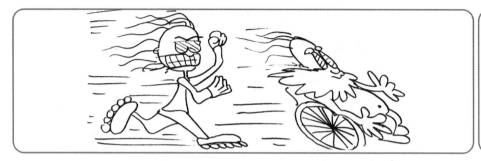

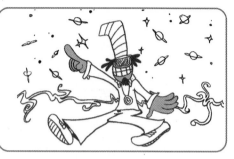

Basic Features Can Be Used in Advanced Ways

You can train a body's ordinary ability into an extraordinary ability.

Here are some things people have trained their bodies to do.

High Performance Mobility

- Kimberly Ames rollerbladed 283 miles in 24 hours in Portland, OR.*

- Rick Hansen, paralyzed from the waist down in a car accident, wheeled his wheelchair 24,901 miles. He went through 4 continents and 34 countries, taking 2 years.

High Performance Language

- Rebel X.D. of Chicago, IL rapped 674 syllables in 54.0 seconds.

- Mike Hessman of Columbus, Ohio told 12,682 jokes in 24 hours.

*Records from **The Guinness Book of World Records**, 1996 edn
World © 1995 Guinness Publishing Ltd
The Guinness Book of World Records is a Trade Mark of Guinness Publishing Ltd

Operator's Manual

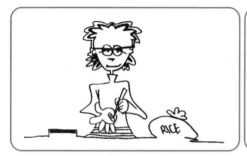

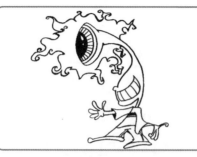

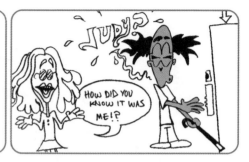

High Performance Manual Coordination

- Om Prakash Singh of Allahabad, India threaded a needle 20,675 times in 2 hours.

- Also in India, Surendra Apharya wrote 1,749 characters on a single grain of rice.

High Performance Vision

- In Houston, Texas, Dr. Dennis M. Levi repeatedly identified the position of a thin, bright green line equivalent to a change of 1/4 inch at a distance of one mile.

High Performance Hearing and Touch

People with visual impairments often demonstrate high performance hearing and touch. Through touch, blind people can read (braille) and recognize facial expressions. They can hear tiny differences and details.

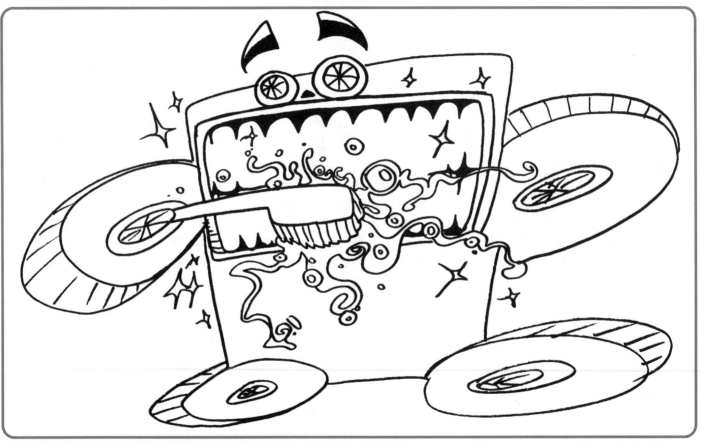

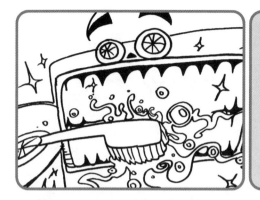

Information about the care of your body is in this section. Health is maintained by using good personal habits.

The body has unlimited energy available if it is maintained correctly.

Energy Maintenance

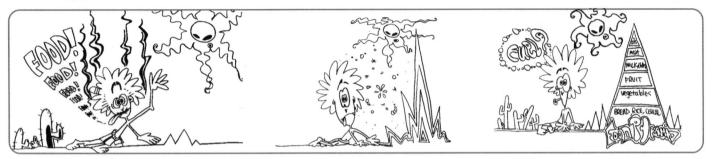

Fuel

Food is your body's fuel and source of energy. For healthy performance, the body needs certain kinds and amounts of food.

The body is equipped with signals to show when it needs food — hunger. You choose the quality and quantity of fuel to consume.

High Performance Fuel

If you eat high performance foods, you will have:

- more energy
- less illness
- fewer cavities
- fewer weight problems.

High performance foods are natural, fresh, and unprocessed.

The Food Guide Pyramid shows a balanced daily diet:

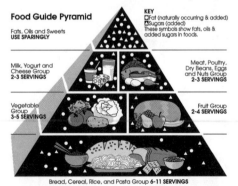

Food Guide Pyramid

Fats, Oils and Sweets
USE SPARINGLY

Milk, Yogurt and Cheese Group
2-3 SERVINGS

Vegetable Group
3-5 SERVINGS

KEY
☐ Fat (naturally occurring & added)
▨ Sugars (added)
These symbols show fats, oils & added sugars in foods.

Meat, Poultry, Dry Beans, Eggs and Nuts Group
2-3 SERVINGS

Fruit Group
2-4 SERVINGS

Bread, Cereal, Rice, and Pasta Group **6-11 SERVINGS**

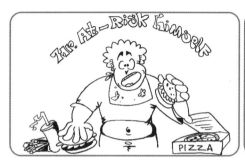

Weak Performance Foods

Foods high in <u>sugar, salt,</u> and <u>oil</u> (junk foods) contain "empty calories." They trick the body into thinking it's been fed — hunger stops, energy is pumped, weight is gained, teeth need brushing — but few or no <u>nutrients</u> actually enter the body!

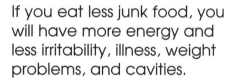

If you eat less junk food, you will have more energy and less irritability, illness, weight problems, and cavities.

Read labels and avoid foods with added sugar (dextrose, etc.) or salt. Put less of these in recipes. Cut back on fats by avoiding fatty meats, whole dairy, nuts, and fried foods.

WARNING!

Minimize consuming artificial sweeteners in foods (in "diet" drinks and "sugarless" foods).

There have been numerous complaints to the FDA about these products.

Energy Maintenance

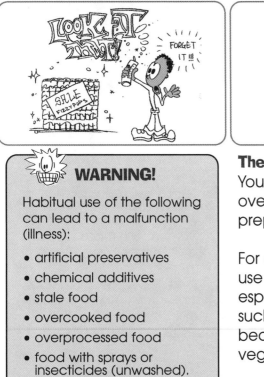

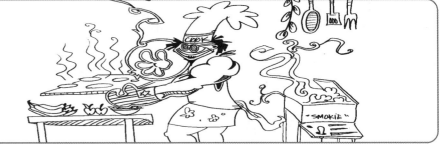

WARNING!

Habitual use of the following can lead to a malfunction (illness):

- artificial preservatives
- chemical additives
- stale food
- overcooked food
- overprocessed food
- food with sprays or insecticides (unwashed).

The Joy of Cooking

You can have more control over what you eat if you prepare it yourself.

For optimum functioning, use <u>fresh</u>, simple foods, especially foods with "fiber," such as whole grains, fruits, beans, peas — and vegetables!

NOTE

Routine attention to kitchen cleanliness and proper storage of foods will prevent food poisoning.

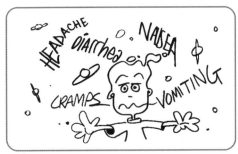

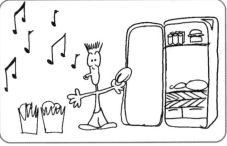

Stop Food Poisoning

Food poisoning is a drag. It feels like the flu. It can kill you. Four ways to avoid it are:

1. <u>Cook It Well</u> Cook meat, poultry, eggs, and seafood thoroughly. Use a meat thermometer.
2. <u>If In Doubt, Throw It Out!</u> This goes for any food that might be spoiled.

3. <u>Keep It Clean</u>
   Always wash your hands before handling food.

   Every time anything (a hand, utensil, or cutting board) touches raw meat, poultry, seafood, or eggs, it must be washed with soap and hot water.

4. <u>Don't Wait...Refrigerate</u>
   Don't leave foods that can spoil (leftovers, pizza, meat, etc.) at room temperature for more than 1-2 hours.

   Here's the rule: Keep hot foods hot (above 140°) and cold foods cold (under 40°).

Energy Maintenance

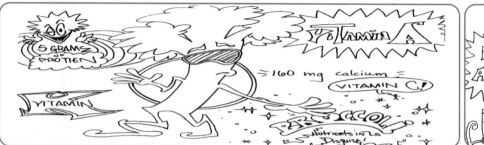 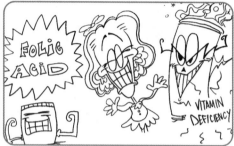

Fuel Mixture

Foods contain vitamins and minerals. The body needs each and every one for a specific purpose. For example, Vitamin A can strengthen vision. Vitamin B can strengthen nerves. Vitamin C builds the immune system and fights infection. Vitamin E is good for your skin.

Minerals have functions, too. For example, calcium builds bones. Iron prevents anemia.

> 👉 **NOTE**
> All women should take <u>folic acid</u> every day during their childbearing years. It helps prevent several birth defects.

The body's vitamin deficiencies show up as symptoms and illnesses. The ideal way to get vitamins and minerals is by eating a variety of fresh, nutritious foods.

Supplements can enhance your diet, but they are not meant to replace healthy food.

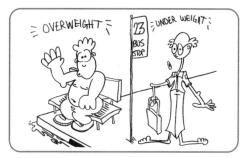

Weigh In

If your body is over or underweight, it cannot work efficiently. If this goes on a long time, the body will react by breaking down, becoming more likely to get a disease or an injury.

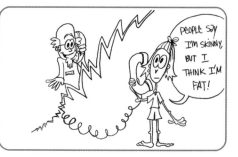

Factors to Weigh

Your body weight also depends on your bone structure, metabolism, and other factors.

If you are concerned about how your weight is affecting your body, consult a health care provider. Don't let it get worse.

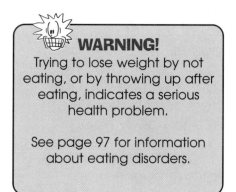

WARNING!

Trying to lose weight by not eating, or by throwing up after eating, indicates a serious health problem.

See page 97 for information about eating disorders.

Energy Maintenance

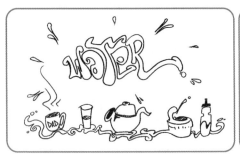

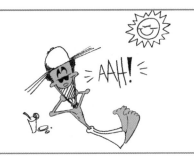

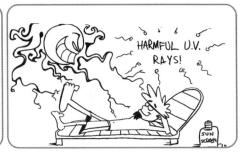

Water

Except for bones and tooth enamel, the body consists mostly (65% - 75%) of water. Water is required for the chemical reactions that keep the body going.

Drink at least 6-8 cups of water throughout an average day; more on hot days. Water is necessary for your body's cooling system.

Breathing

Even though breathing is an automatic function of your body, <u>consciously</u> breathing more deeply will enhance health. Deep breaths provide extra oxygen to the body, helping it deal with all forms of stress and other operations. Breathe <u>clean</u> air as much as possible.

Sunshine

The sun is a source of energy for the body. Get "sun kissed" daily.

WARNING!
Suntans and sunburns can cause skin cancer. Use sun block (SPF 15 or greater). Tans are popular, but not necessarily healthy.

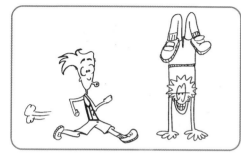

It's the Plan
Your body needs movement. Exercise gives the body:
- cardiovascular fitness
- muscle bulk & strength
- calcium for the bones
- increased oxygen capacity
- flexibility
- the ability to fight illness and deal with stress.

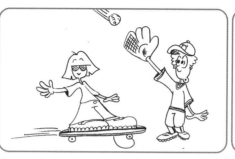

Move It!
Pick something you like: walking, running, skating, swimming, dancing, biking, team sports, etc.

You'll get:
- more energy
- less flab
- better sleep
- better appetite
- clearer thinking.

Use it or Lose It
Your body needs the equivalent of at least <u>30 minutes</u> of exercise <u>3 times a week</u>. Each time: warm up, get aerobic, stretch and strengthen, and cool down.

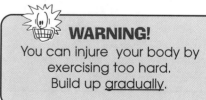

WARNING!
You can injure your body by exercising too hard.
Build up <u>gradually</u>.

Energy Maintenance

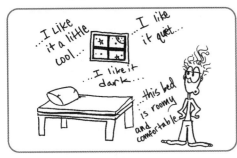

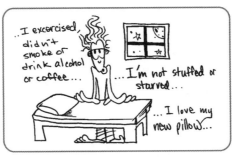

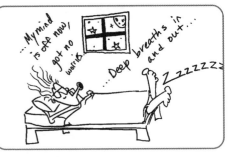

Bodies Need Sleep

Human bodies require 5 - 10 hours of sleep every 24 hours (most people need 7 - 8 hours). Sleep gives the body energy and mental clarity.

> ☞ **NOTE**
> Cells regenerate during sleep. Dreams release tension and can give you insights about yourself.

Get a Routine

It is healthiest to sleep at the same time every day or night.

Your body is equipped with signals that tell you it needs rest (quick loss of body strength or concentration). If you feel tired, take a nap during the day. If you deprive your body of sleep, catch up.

Sleep Troubles

If you often have trouble sleeping, get professional help, not pills.

> **WARNING!**
> Overriding the "tired" signal with a stimulant, such as coffee, will eventually lead to a breakdown of body functioning and illness.

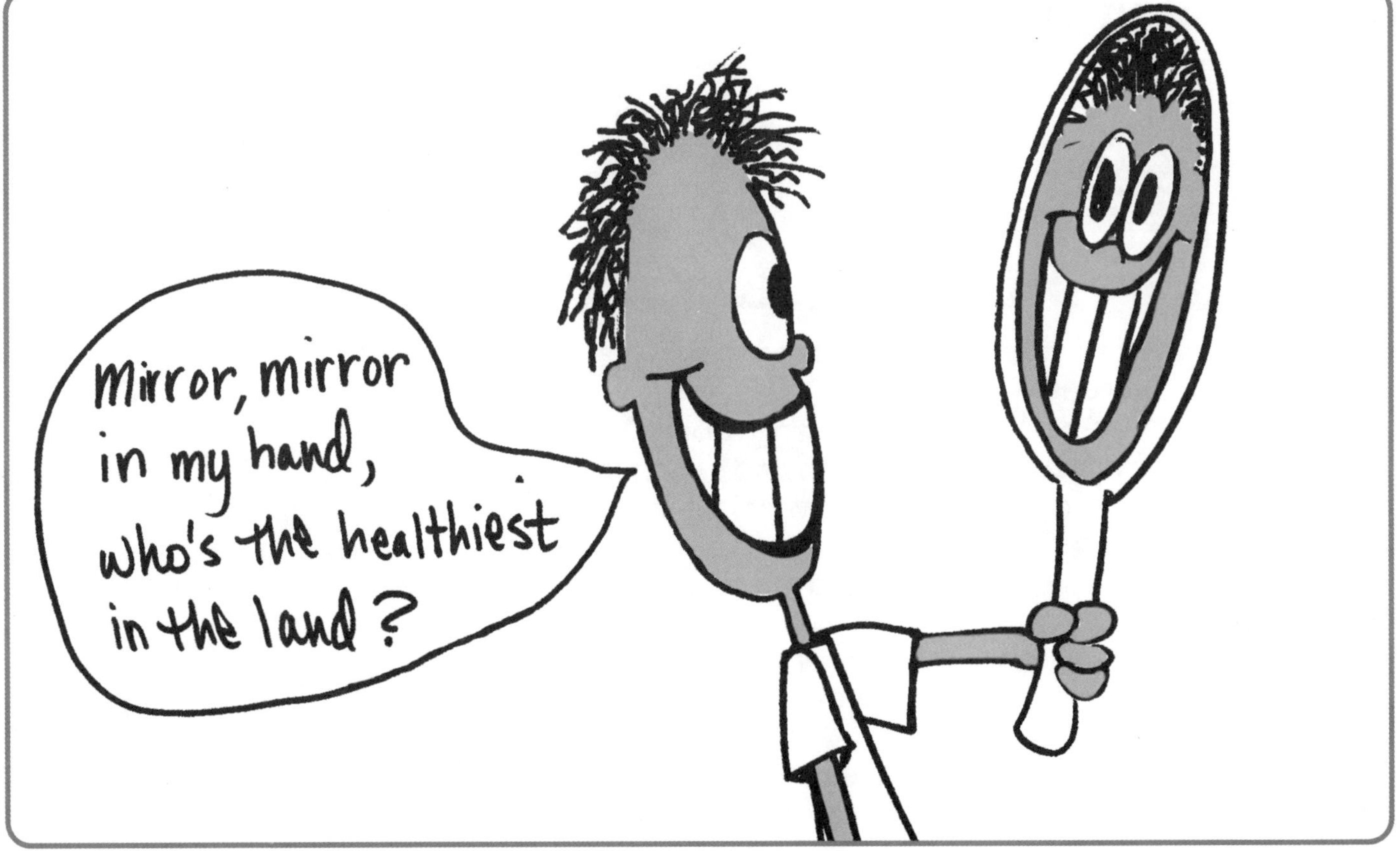
Mirror, mirror in my hand, who's the healthiest in the land?

Eye Maintenance

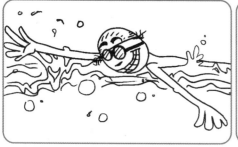

One Set per Customer
The windows (eyes) on your vehicle are very difficult to repair and replace, so special maintenance is required.

Wear protective glasses or goggles during these activities:

- sports (to avoid impact)

- cleaning, painting, lab work, and swimming (to avoid chemicals)

- grinding, sawing and cutting (to avoid getting bits of materials in the eyes)

- welding and activities involving fire.

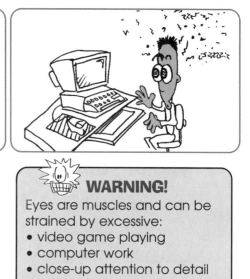

WARNING!
Eyes are muscles and can be strained by excessive:
- video game playing
- computer work
- close-up attention to detail (e.g., sewing)
- prolonged driving
- extreme contrasts, such as looking at a computer monitor or watching TV in a dark room.

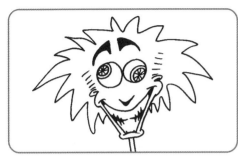

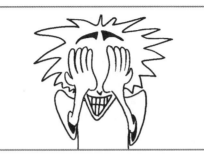

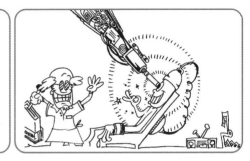

Eye Care (Don't You?)

Your eyes need exercise, just like the other muscles in your body. Some activities that improve the health of the eyes are to:

- Move eyes up, down, and side to side. Blink often.

- Avoid staring, rubbing, and squinting.

- Rest eyes from close work by focusing far away, then close up several times.

- Rest eyes from looking at a light source by "palming" (placing the palms of the hands over the eyes). Breathe and relax.

See an Eye Doctor

Make an appointment with an eye doctor if your eyes:

- hurt
- itch
- seem irritated
- don't see clearly.

If you wear glasses, see an eye doctor regularly.

Exterior Maintenance

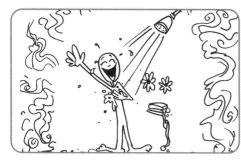

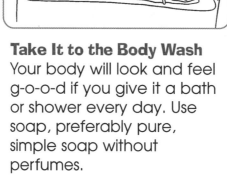

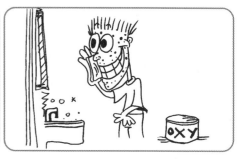

Hygiene Routines

You are responsible for taking care of the exterior of your body.

You can prevent illness by washing. Also, if you don't wash, the buildup of bacteria will cause you to stink.

Take It to the Body Wash

Your body will look and feel g-o-o-d if you give it a bath or shower every day. Use soap, preferably pure, simple soap without perfumes.

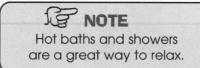

☞ **NOTE**
Hot baths and showers are a great way to relax.

Skin Maintenance

If your body was manufactured 12-20 years ago, you will probably notice your skin sprouting pimples. If your skin has many pimples that persist, it's called acne.

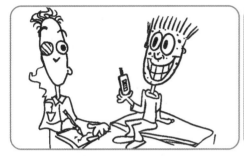

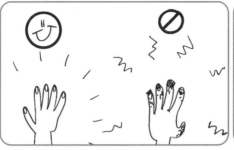

More on Less Acne

The best way to deal with acne is to keep your skin free of dirt, oil, and sweat. Wash your skin gently. Avoid rubbing, squeezing, or picking pimples.

Cosmetics can aggravate acne by clogging skin pores. Use "non-comedogenic" make-up.

Claw Maintenance

Because of the way nails are structured, dirt tends to collect around and under them.

To make a good impression on a potential employer, or a date, or anyone, keep your nails clean and trimmed.

Nail Biting

Nail biting is a nervous habit. If you need help in stopping:

- Use "Nail Biter" nail polish (tastes bad), or
- Wear a rubber band that fits comfortably around your wrist. Every time you think of biting, pull on the rubber band and give yourself a small stinging reminder not to.

Exterior Maintenance

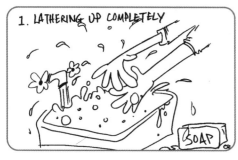

1. LATHERING UP COMPLETELY

SOAP

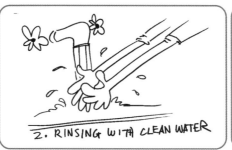

2. RINSING WITH CLEAN WATER

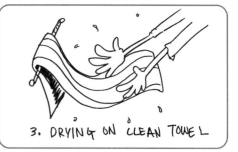

3. DRYING ON CLEAN TOWEL

The Hands Routine
Hands are the most common way infections are spread. To prevent illness, wash your hands:

- after using the bathroom
- after changing a diaper
- after sneezing
- after touching raw meat
- before cooking/eating
- after touching cat litter.

The Hands Wash
To remove bacteria when washing hands:

1. Use warm water.
2. Use soap (preferably liquid, which hasn't touched others' hands).
3. Rub soap all over hands, working up a lather (about 20 seconds).

4. Rinse hands in clean, running water.
5. Dry hands on a clean or paper towel.
6. In a public bathroom, you may want to use the towel to turn off the water and turn the doorknob.

 NOTE
If your hands are dry, rub some lotion on them.

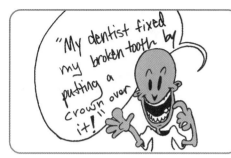

Smile!

A healthy-looking mouth requires daiy maintenance and periodic visits to a dentist to spot and fix problems.

> ☞ **NOTE**
> If you don't have a dentist, ask a friend to recommend one.

Fang Maintenance

A healthy diet creates stronger teeth. Brush and floss after eating to avoid cavities. Use a toothpaste that contains fluoride to help prevent cavities.

> **WARNING!**
> Whiteners in toothpaste actually remove tiny layers of enamel. Go easy! Use only occasionally.

Brushing works by removing bits of food before they combine with the bacteria that live in the mouth to make acid. Acid eats through the enamel coating of the tooth, making a cavity.

Built-up food and bacteria create plaque, stain teeth, and can cause gum disease and bad breath.

Exterior Maintenance

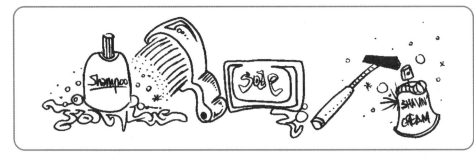

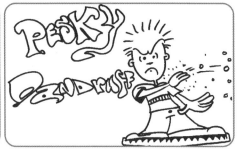

The Hair Routine

Maintain your hair by washing it with shampoo often enough to avoid greasiness. Brush and comb it daily. Having it cut periodically keeps your hair healthy.

WARNING!

Hair treatments such as dying, straightening, and perming have chemicals that may damage your hair.

Be sure to follow the product's directions and read warnings.

Pesky Dandruff

If your scalp isn't itchy, but small white flakes of dry skin are showering down from it, you've probably got dandruff.

If it's not too bad, you can take care of it by following the directions on an anti-dandruff shampoo.

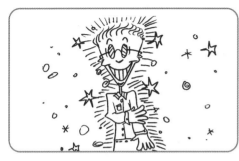

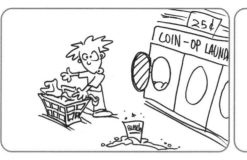

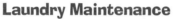

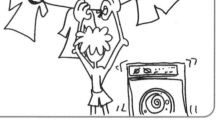

Suds 'n' Duds Hygiene

No matter what style of clothing you choose to wear, it's important for health reasons to keep it clean.

> ☞ **NOTE**
>
> Have at least two sets of clothes, towels, and bedding so there is always a clean set ready.

Laundry Maintenance

1. Deal with stains right when they happen; scrub off with soap and water (cold for blood; hot for others).

2. Avoid the pink T-shirt syndrome. Sort white/lights and color/darks, and wash them separately.

3. Get things out of the dryer right away. As you fold them, rub out the wrinkles. Put clothes on hangers to avoid wrinkles.

4. Change bedding and towels about once a week.

Interior Maintenance

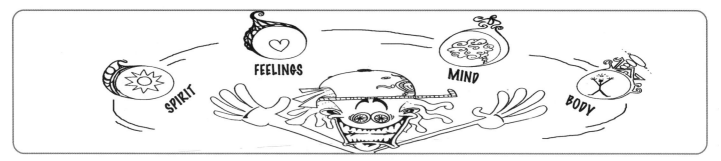

Staying Balanced

Your system drives along on four points of balance:

> BODY
> MIND
> FEELINGS
> SPIRIT

If you neglect any of these, it's like letting the air out of a tire; you'll have a bumpy ride.

Know Your Sides

This operator's manual concentrates on the BODY, or physical point of balance. But there are three others:

— Your MIND is an exceptional tool that needs to be continually sharpened by thinking, learning, and interacting with others.

— FEELINGS come from your heart and steer you through the path of life. You don't always have to act on your feelings, but it's healthy to know them.

— Your SPIRITUAL side is your sense of purpose, creativity, intuition, and connection with a life force.

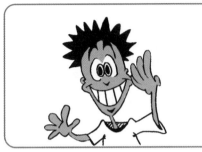

Self-Esteem

Self-esteem is your own opinion of yourself; not anyone else's. To build self-esteem, observe your thoughts, feelings, and actions, and accept yourself as you are.

If you see something in yourself you don't like, the mind is equipped to change it.

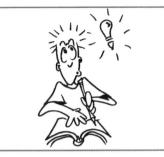

Self-Responsibility

Many things may happen in your life over which you have little or no control. How you respond is a personal choice. It is more helpful to see how you have chosen to handle a situation than to look for someone to blame.

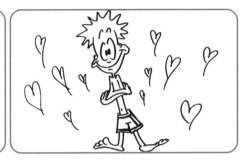

Self-Care

Self-care means doing the things that give you pleasure (without hurting yourself or others). Take time to do the things that you really enjoy. Fun is food for the soul.

Interior Maintenance

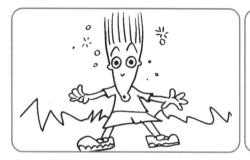

Emotional Support (Help!)

Being human is confusing. It is natural to want to find a way around this confused state. Share your thoughts and feelings with a friend. If you're really stuck, talk to a counselor. Ask around. Find someone you can relate to.

Finding a Good Counselor

Exercise your freedom of choice when it comes to counselors. After a few sessions, you can tell if someone:

- is trustworthy
- can understand you
- really cares about you
- listens compassionately
- has the skill to help you make changes.

> ☞ **NOTE**
> Even if you are assigned a counselor, you still have a choice about whom you want to work with. Don't be shy; ask about your options.

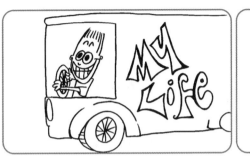

Cruise Control

Stresses and emotions impact on your system. Keep your internal state running smoothly by defusing the stress and emotions before they build up.

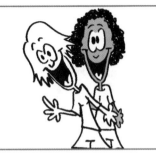

Healthy Pleasures

People maintain their inner health through:

- sports or exercise
- meditation and breathing
- reading
- writing in a journal
- being in nature
- hobbies
- helping others.

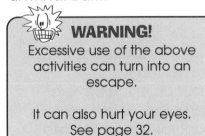

Monitor Yourself

TV, video games, and net surfing can be fun ways to unwind. But...

WARNING!
Excessive use of the above activities can turn into an escape.

It can also hurt your eyes. See page 32.

Social Maintenance

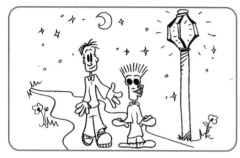

Reaching Out

"Everybody needs somebody sometimes." Do you have someone you can:

- talk to about anything?
- have fun with?
- call on if you have a problem or are upset?
- ask for help with child care (if you're a parent)?
- visit or who visits you?
- ask for help with things like house repairs?
- talk to about big decisions?

Friendship is a two-way street. Be sure you're there when people reach out to you.

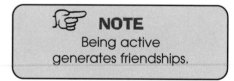

NOTE
Being active generates friendships.

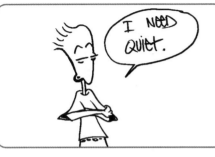

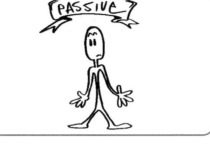

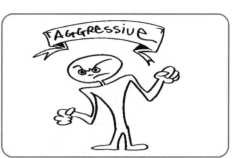

Tuned-Up Communication

Be <u>assertive</u>. Ask for what you want or need in a simple and direct way.

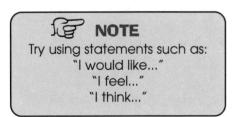

NOTE

Try using statements such as:
"I would like..."
"I feel..."
"I think..."

When you don't state what you want or need — and are too <u>passive</u>, you give up your right to make a choice.

On the other hand, if you are too <u>aggressive</u>, you impose your ideas on others and destroy the chance to have their input.

<u>Passive-aggressive</u> actions are when a person doesn't state his or her need but does something (hurtful) that shows it.

Examples are putting things off, being late, "forgetting" work, or being sulky when someone asks you to do something you don't want to do.

Social Maintenance

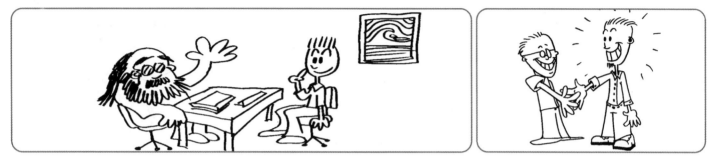

Manners

Manners are cultural rules for acceptable behavior in social situations. Most of these are not laws but help people live together in peace.

If you going to a job interview, for example, here are some manners to use:

- Stand face-to-face; not too close; not too far away.
- Shake hands; not too loose, not too tight.
- Make eye contact; not too little, not too much.

- Speak clearly; not too loud, not too soft.
- Dress up; not too much, not too little.
- Sit up straight; not too little, not too much.
- Give answers; not too short, not too long.

Manners are learned by watching good role models.

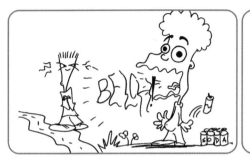

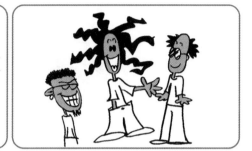

Be Aware!
Here are some habits that others may find annoying:
- belching
- farting
- spitting
- swearing
- picking your nose
- picking at scabs
- excessive scratching
- cracking knuckles
- nervous tapping.

Amazing Grace
Here are some ways to make others feel good:

- using positive language
- using a soft tone of voice
- listening politely
- responding to others' feelings and needs
- expressing appreciation
- following through with a promise.

WARNING!
When you choose to express yourself in socially different ways, it may slow you down from getting what you want.

Environmental Maintenance

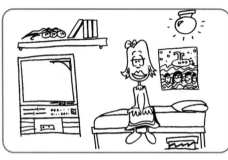

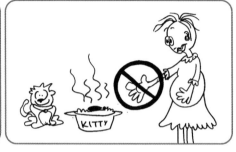

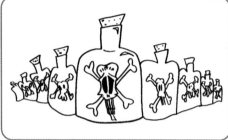

Home Sweet Home
Your home is the environment you create for yourself. Keeping it clean and organized cuts your chances of getting sick.

Be sure that your room:
- Has good fresh-air ventilation.
- Is free of dust and dirt.

WARNING!
Women who are or plan to get pregnant should not touch the litter box (feces) of a cat, or they could get toxoplasmosis.

Household Poisons
Be sure to check labels to see if your household products, like cleaners, are poisonous. Store poisons in places that are out of reach from children and away from foods.

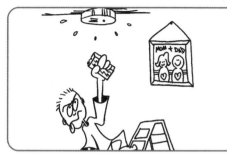

Don't Get Burned

Part of maintaining your home environment is to practice fire safety and prevention. Here's how:

1. Make sure you have an updated smoke alarm. The better ones have a 10-year life battery. Check it regularly.

2. Know your exit plan in case of fire.

3. Make sure the windows and gratings open for emergency exit.

4. Keep a fire extinguisher and/or baking soda available in your kitchen.

5. Put out grease fires with baking soda, not water.

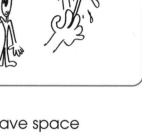

6. Don't leave space heaters on when no one is home.

7. If you smoke, don't do it in bed.

8. Put out matches and cigarettes thoroughly.

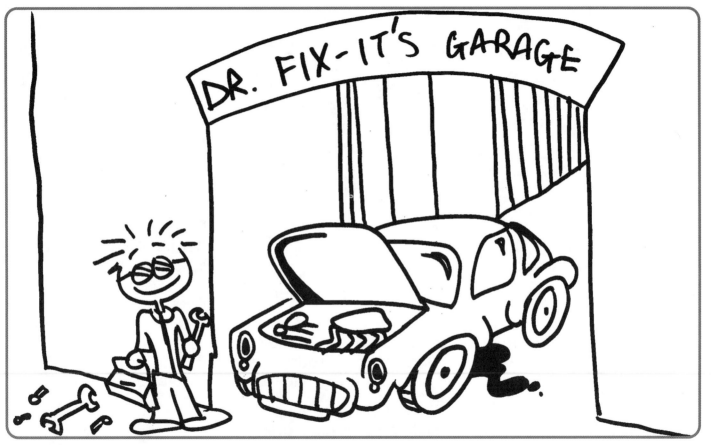

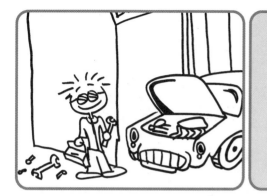

Your body will require repairs periodically.

This section will help you know what to do.

Warning Signs

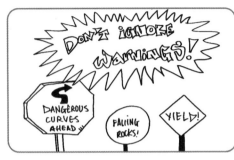

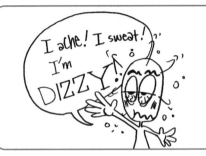

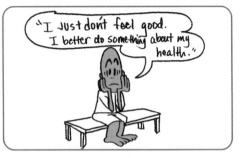

Symptoms are Signs

Your body comes with a warning system to let you know when it needs special attention.

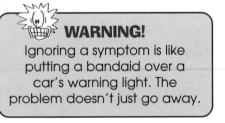

WARNING!

Ignoring a symptom is like putting a bandaid over a car's warning light. The problem doesn't just go away.

Red Alert Symptoms

Symptoms are sensations that don't feel good.

Some obvious symptoms are:

- aches and pains
- coughing or sneezing
- fever
- sores
- dizziness
- anything "strange."

Caution Symptoms

If you are feeling:
- tired
- cranky
- withdrawn,

it also means that your body is saying, "Do something." Think about why you feel this way and try to solve the problem.

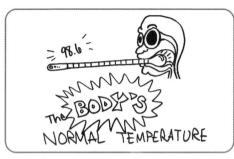

Body Temperature

98.6°F - 99.6°F is "normal," i.e., healthy. Less than 97.6°F may be due to a virus. More than 99.6°F means you have a fever.

Call a nurse if a fever is higher than 101°F.

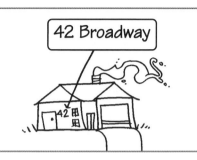

Advance Preparations

Prepare for emergencies by knowing who, when, how to call, and what to do until help arrives.

- Keep emergency numbers by the phone.
- Be sure your house or apartment number is easily seen.

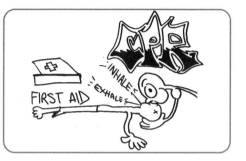

- Keep a copy of your medical history handy.
- Keep a First Aid kit and know how to use it.
- Have a copy of the Red Cross **First Aid** book. Look through it.
- Learn CPR; know how to handle choking and serious bleeding.

Make a Plan

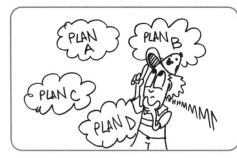 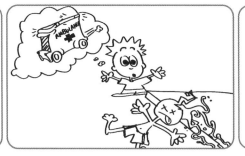 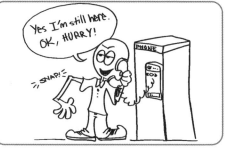

Make a Plan

Paying attention to the body's warning signals means choosing one of these plans:

A. Call an **A**mbulance
B. **B**uzz over to the emergency room
C. **C**all the doctor
D. **D**ial Ask-a-Nurse
E. **E**ducate yourself with a medical reference book.

Plan A:
Call an Ambulance!

Medical emergencies include:
- *choking*
- *severe burns*
- *bleeding you can't stop*
- *extreme chest pain*
- *seizures*
- *very high fever*
- *blacking out*
- *incoherence* (from poisoning or overdose)

Call 9-1-1

In a medical emergency, call 911 and ask for an ambulance. Be ready to tell them your name, phone number, and address (directions, landmarks). State what is happening. Answer questions, and **DON'T HANG UP UNTIL YOU'RE TOLD TO!**

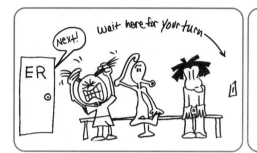

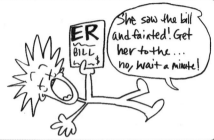

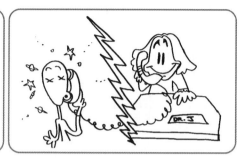

Plan B:
Buzz Over to the ER

Go or have someone take you to the emergency room for conditions that are urgent but not immediately life-threatening, such as a deep cut that doesn't spurt blood or simple fracture.

Don't go to the ER if you can make an appointment with your doctor instead or fix the problem some other way.

ER visits are <u>expensive</u>, both in time and money!

Plan C:
Call the Doctor

Call your doctor's office to find out whether you need to see a doctor or treat yourself with over-the-counter medications and/or First Aid.

Make a Plan

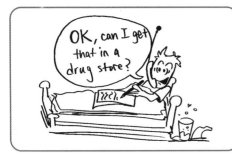

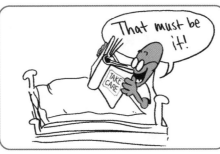

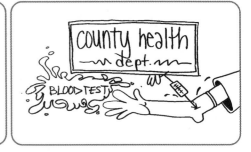

Plan D:
Dial Ask-a-Nurse
Most places have an Ask-a-Nurse program which you can call and receive free medical information. Nurses cannot diagnose your problem over the phone, but they can tell you if you should be examined by a doctor or take care of it yourself.

Plan E:
Educate Yourself
It's a good idea to own a copy of a medical reference book like **Take Care of Yourself**. When you have symptoms, you can use the book to find out what might be going on and what to do about it. For titles of other good health books, see **Read Up!** on p. 166.

> ☞ **NOTE**
> You can get tests and shots at the County Public Health Department. Find it in the "County" section of the government pages in the telephone book.
>
> Call first to find out what tests/shots you can get there (e.g., HIV testing, immunizations, etc.).

Health Care Providers

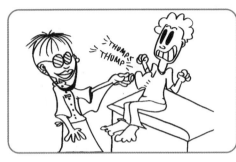

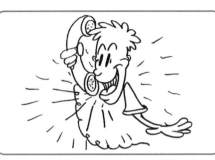

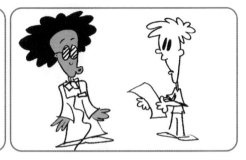

Choosing Doctors
When you choose medical care givers, consider:

- their ability/willingness to answer your questions
- the type of care you want (conventional, holistic, etc.)
- convenience (location).

Dealing with Doctors
- Make an appointment.
- Show up on time or call ahead (at least 24 hours).
- Be ready to answer medical history questions.
- If you have symptoms, this is the time to discuss them. Remember when they started, what they've been like, and what you've done for them.

- Make a list of questions that you want to ask the doctor and bring it.
- If you feel uneasy with a doctor's decision/advice, get a second opinion.

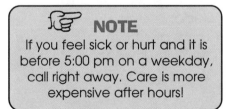

☞ **NOTE**
If you feel sick or hurt and it is before 5:00 pm on a weekday, call right away. Care is more expensive after hours!

Common Problems

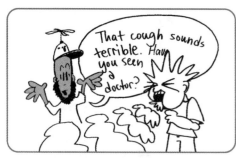

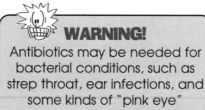

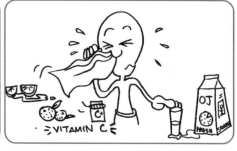

Bacterial Infections

You may have a bacterial infection if you have...

- fever above 99.6°F
- increased pain, redness, and/or swelling after the second day
- thick pus from a wound or thick sputum (spit) when you cough.

If you think you have a bacterial infection, see a doctor.

WARNING!

Antibiotics may be needed for bacterial conditions, such as strep throat, ear infections, and some kinds of "pink eye" (conjunctivitis).
Consult a doctor.

Colds

The common cold is a virus that inflames your lungs and sinuses. Treat it with rest, lots of liquids, and vitamin C. If it lasts longer than a week or it gets worse, call a doctor.

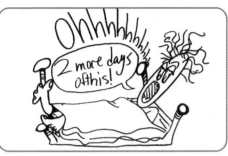

Flu

If you think you are getting the flu (muscle aches, fever, vomiting, diarrhea), call a medical professional. Describe your symptoms. S/he can tell you if it's "that bug that's going around" and how long it'll probably last.

Headaches

Many headaches are caused by tension. The solution is to relax. Close your eyes. Drink more water. Breathe more deeply. Increase circulation with neck rolls and massage.

You also can get a headache from excess hunger and fatigue.

If a headache persists, you can take acetaminophen or ibuprofen (e.g., Tylenol or Advil). Taking aspirin can cause Reye's Syndrome, a serious health problem.

If a headache comes with fever, nausea, pus in your ears, or trouble seeing — call a doctor.

Common Problems

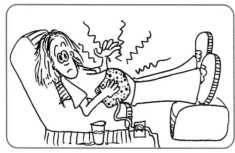

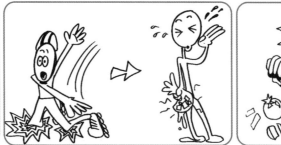

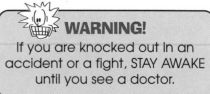

Menstrual Cramps

For teenage women, it is common to feel discomfort during the monthly period.

Cramps can be eased by exercise, heat (hot water bottle or heating pad) applied to the lower abdomen, or by taking ibuprofen.

Minor Injuries

Everybody gets minor cuts, scrapes, burns, bites, bumps, and sprains. If you are treating a minor injury at home, remember to:

- keep wounds clean
- use ice to keep swelling down
- not put weight on anything that hurts.

Consult a medical reference book, such as the Red Cross **First Aid** book.

If pain continues, call a doctor or Ask-a-Nurse.

WARNING!
If you are knocked out in an accident or a fight, STAY AWAKE until you see a doctor.

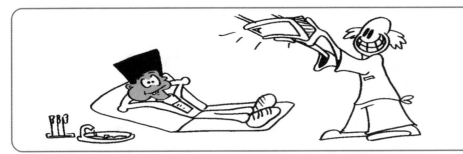

Mouth Problems

Your adult teeth should last a lifetime. Don't let them get stained, chipped, or pulled unless it's absolutely necessary.

Your mouth is exposed and vulnerable to germs. If germs get out of control in your mouth, you can get:

- tooth pain
- bleeding gums
- sores.

If this happens, see a dentist immediately.

Sore Throats

Swollen glands, soreness, and rash can be part of a sore throat. Use a flashlight to see if there are white splotches (pus pockets) in the back of your mouth. If you have these or any severe or prolonged symptoms, see a doctor. Meanwhile, gargle with warm water and ¼ teaspoon salt.

Common Problems

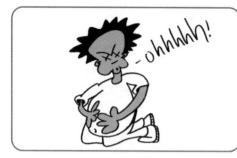

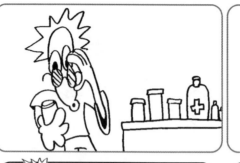

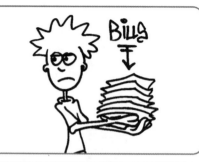

Stomach Aches

Stomach aches can mean many things — anxiety, stress, indigestion, female problems... and more serious conditions, such as appendicitis.

If a stomach ache seems severe or hangs on a long time, call for help.

WARNING!

- Don't take other people's pills.
- Don't take outdated pills.
- Take all pills <u>as prescribed</u>.
- Read all labels.
- Never mix pills with alcohol or drugs!

NOTE

Since you never know when you are going to get an injury or illness, it is important to always have access to medical care.

Medical care is very expensive. Always carry medical insurance.

Invasions

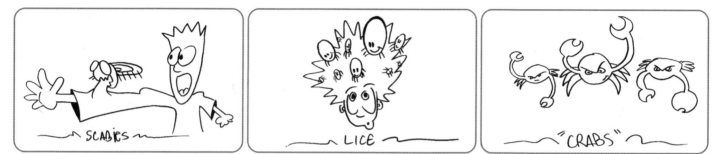

Scabies, Head Lice, and Crabs

People can get these very itchy critters by being in contact with someone else who has them — or their clothes or bedding.

Scabies are mites that burrow under the skin on your hands or in your skin creases, leaving red lines.

Lice like to live in hair. You can see their "nits" (eggs) as tiny white lumps which "stick" more than dandruff. Lice in pubic hair are called "crabs."

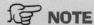 **NOTE**
Head lice are spread by using other people's hairbrushes or combs.

What to Do

If you think you might have an invasion happening, get checked by a health care provider immediately. There's medicine to take and washing to do. Be sure to tell people you've had contact with.

Stress

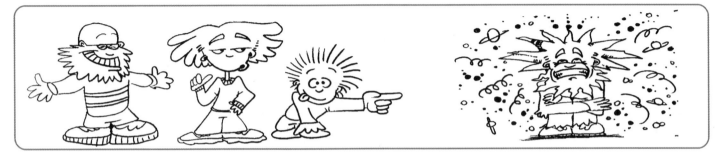

Stress

Stress usually comes from fear and anxiety. Ignoring or abusing the body's needs can also produce stress.

Stress can produce many different symptoms, such as nervous habits, headaches, migraines, stomach aches, and fatigue.

Being stressed can lead to making poor decisions, because you might not think things all the way through.

Stress Habits

Sometimes stress shows itself as physical habits. Some of the most common are:

- fingernail biting
- teeth clenching
- smoking
- repeated motions, such as finger tapping or leg twitching.

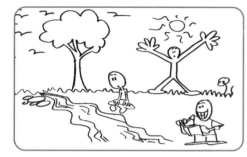 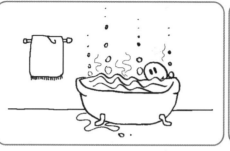 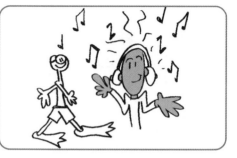

Stress Relief

To relieve stress, do some of these:

- Take deep breaths.
- Exercise, take a walk.
- Think, write, or talk about what's bothering you.
- Make a plan.
- Talk to a counselor.
- Cry.

To just loosen up, try:

- taking a hot bath
- reading a magazine
- calling a friend
- listening to music
- taking a break — short or long.

WARNING !
Taking pills may seem to cover up the discomforts of stress, but this won't get to the root of the problem, where it can be solved.

Anger

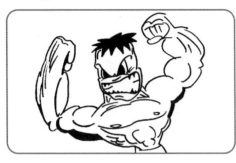

Grrrrr!
Frustration at not getting what you want — whether it is right or wrong — builds anger.

Getting Angry
Sure signs that you are angry are when:

- People tell you that you are raising your voice.

- You feel like hitting someone.

- Your body is tense.

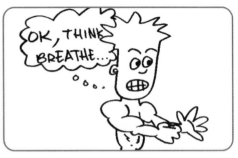

Two Choices
If you are angry, you can <u>let it grow</u> or <u>slow it down</u>.

To slow it down:
- Pull away.
- Slowly count to ten.
- Redirect the angry energy in a safe way.
- Think it out.
- Give it time.
- Try a new approach toward a solution.

Operator's Manual

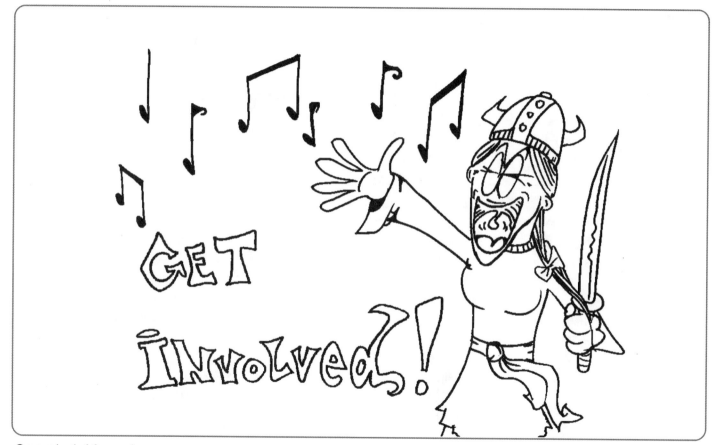

Depression

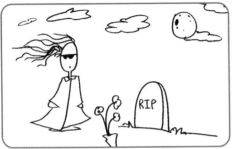

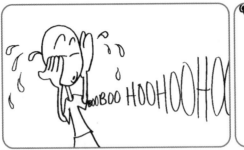

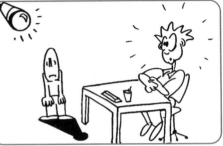

Down Time

There are many levels of feeling down, from everyday blues to serious depression.

Everyone gets the blues. It's natural to feel sad, especially when you've lost something or had a disappointment.

Light Blues

Light blues come and go. If your blues come with tears, go ahead and cry. Did you know that chemicals released in tears have a calming effect?

Sometimes relaxing will help get you through the light blues. Learn what works for you.

Dark Blues

If you can't snap out of the blues, talk about your situation with a counselor.

If any of the following signs persist, you may need to get help:

- getting way too little or too much sleep — or food
- feeling tired all the time

Operator's Manual

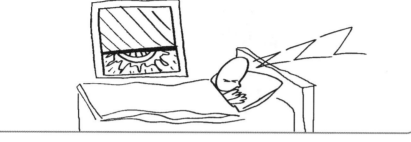

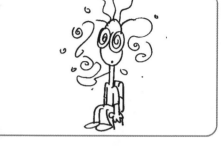

Signs of depression, continued

- having trouble getting things done
- having trouble thinking clearly or concentrating
- staying away from people
- feeling uninterested; nothing's fun
- feeling irritable and/or angry a lot
- feeling slow and restless

- feeling hopeless and helpless
- crying a lot
- feeling sorry for yourself
- feeling suicidal.

WARNING!
If you have a plan to take your life, call a suicide hotline or go to the nearest emergency room <u>right away</u>.

NOTE
If you are taking medication, check with your doctor to see if a side effect of the medication is depression.

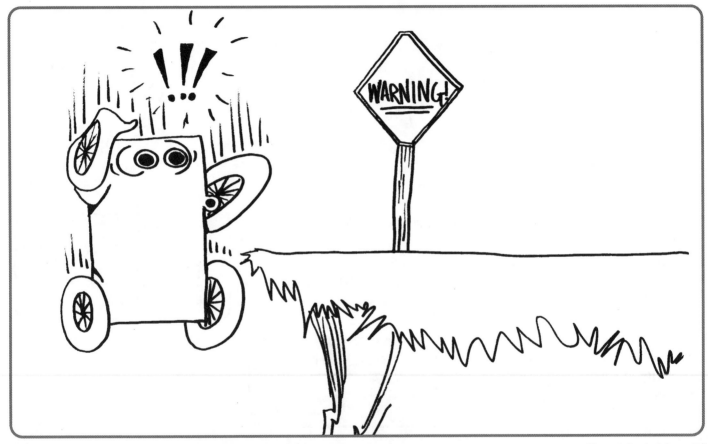

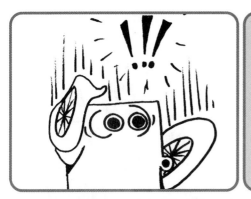

Here's information about how — and why — you should steer clear of these dangers on the road of life.

Accidents

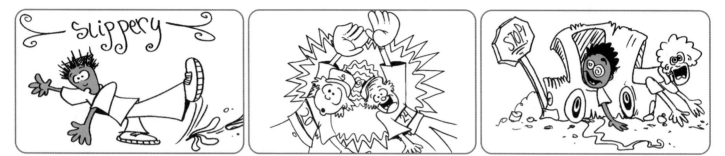

The 7 Most Common Non-Fatal Injuries of the Teen Body (in order)

1. falls

2. being hit by an object (in crowds, during sports, by falling objects)

3. motor vehicle accidents

4. overexertion or strenuous movement (sports-related)

5. cutting and piercing

6. natural or environmental factors (hypo- or hyper-thermia, changes in air pressure, lack of food or water, animal bites, lightning, earthquakes, tornadoes, etc.)

7. fire or flames.

Information obtained from Centers for Disease Control.

Operator's Manual

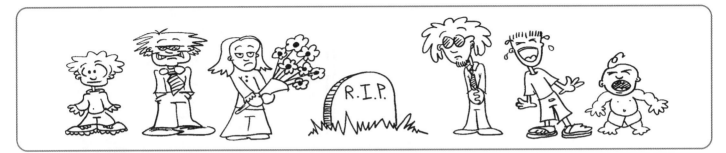

The 9 Most Common Fatal Injuries of the Teen Body (in order)

1. motor vehicle accidents

2. homicide by firearms

3. suicide by firearms

4. suicide by suffocation

5. unintentional drowning

6. unintentional poisoning

7. homicide by cutting or piercing

8. firearm accidents

9. suicide by poisoning.

Information obtained from Centers for Disease Control.

Safety

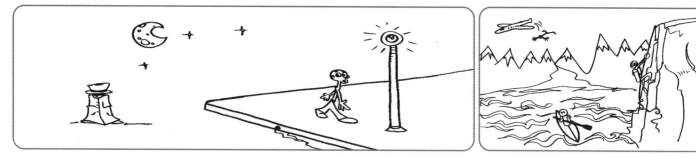

Classic Safety Tips

- Stay on the light side of the street and where there are people.

- Trust your judgment, don't ride or talk with people if it doesn't feel right.

- Carry only money you need, in a secure pocket.

- Carry emergency phone numbers and special medical information in your wallet.

- For longer visits, make sure that someone at your destination knows when you're coming.

Calculated Risks

The way to avoid accidents is to <u>Think First</u> and <u>Be Prepared</u>. Ask yourself:

- Are my skills up for this?
- Is the weather right?
- Is my equipment safe?

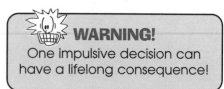

WARNING!
One impulsive decision can have a lifelong consequence!

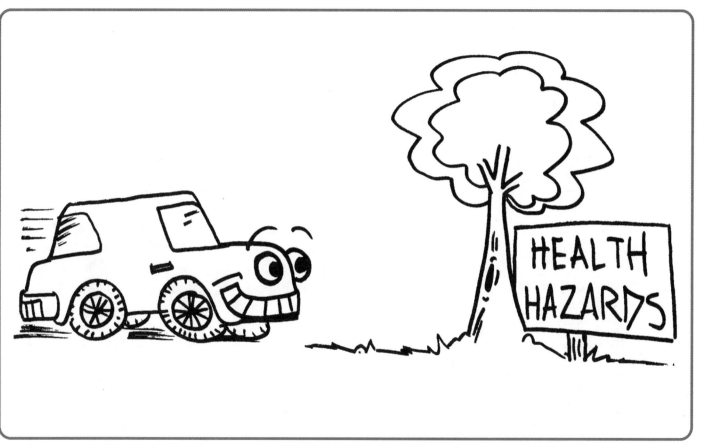

Alcohol

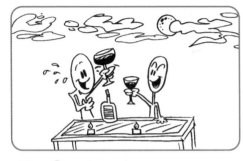

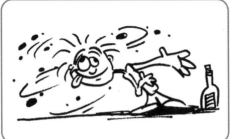

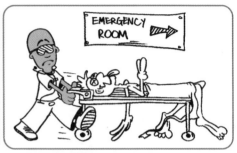

The Good
Alcohol can, in small amounts, improve circulation, reduce blood pressure and be relaxing.

> 👉 **NOTE**
> In most places, there are legal restrictions to having alcohol if you are under 21.

The Bad
Drinking alcohol is a problem for millions of people. Alcoholism is a disease that can happen at any age. If there is alcoholism in your birth family, you are more susceptible to problem drinking. This is especially true for girls.

The Ugly
- Alcohol overdose is the #1 drug-related case seen in hospital emergency rooms.

- Alcohol is the #1 cause of car accidents.

- Alcohol can cause bad thinking and judgment.

- Alcohol may interfere with healthy eating and nutrition.

Operator's Manual

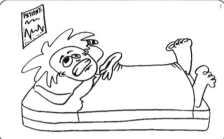

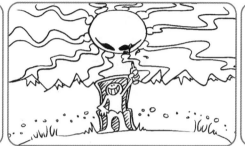

- Alcohol can cause permanent damage to the body.
- Alcohol contributes to the occurrence of unwanted pregnancies.
- Alcohol can cause permanent damage to the fetus during pregnancy.

Clues

Alcohol is a problem for you if you:

- drink to deal with feeling bad
- have trouble remembering what happened when you were drunk
- drink even after you decide to stay sober
- drink early in the day
- miss class or work because you are hung over
- drink to feel comfortable with people.

Illegal Drugs

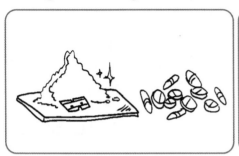

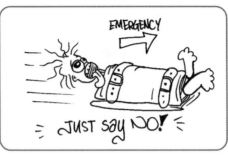

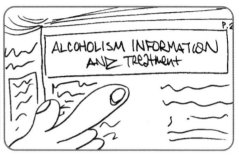

Personal Choices

Illegal drugs produce a variety of sensations, but there are also well-known problems caused by using illegal drugs, such as:

- addiction
- illness and disease
- permanent injury or death
- money problems
- legal problems

- emotional problems
- relationship problems
- employment problems
- school problems.

Every teen has to make a choice between short-term drug experiences and the reality of long-term damage.

Getting Help for Drug or Alcohol Problems

Many different treatments are available for substance abuse problems. Contact information is available through the Yellow Pages, under "Alcoholism Information and Treatment" or "Drug Abuse Information and Treatment."

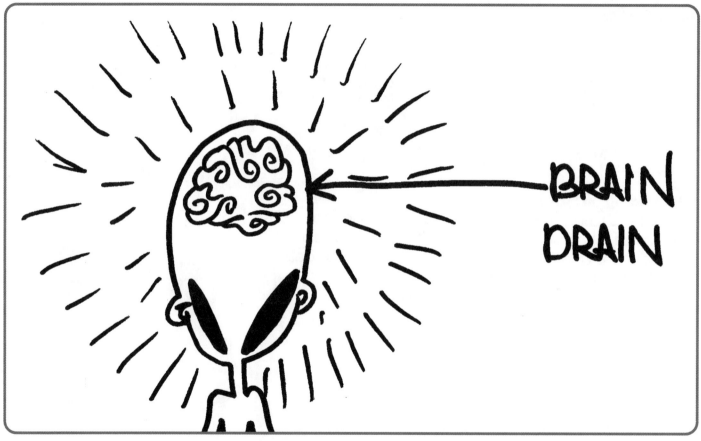

Caffeine

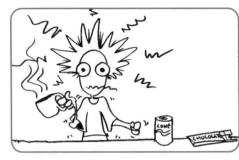

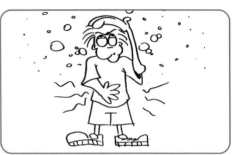

Depending on Stim?

Caffeine is found in coffee, tea, colas, chocolate, some medications and most weight loss aids. Most people feel more energetic after having it, for about 30 minutes.

Excess caffeine may cause the jitters, poor sleep, a racing heart, headaches, or stomach upset, and it stains your teeth.

WARNING!

If you drink over 3 cups of coffee a day, you may be dependent on caffeine.

If you suddenly go without it, you may experience withdrawal symptoms (headache, fatigue, irritability, depression).

Tobacco

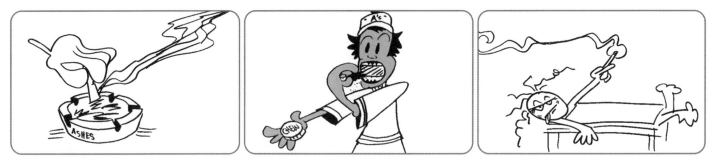

The Smoking Gun
Nicotine in cigarettes and chewing tobacco is highly addictive. One in every five persons in the U.S. will die from diseases caused by smoking or chewing.

"Quitting cigarettes isn't hard at all. Why, I've done it 23 times!"

— Mark Twain (adapted)

Germs and Diseases

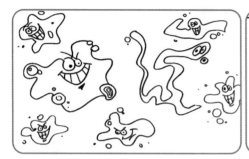

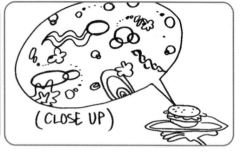

Germs: They're There

Germs are everywhere. Some are friendly to the human body. Those that are unhealthy for the human body can be controlled by knowing how they spread.

Germ Transportation

Germs spread disease in four ways:

1. **Breathing.** Germs that cause colds, flu, strep throat, meningitis, and chicken pox ride on sneezes, coughs, and spit (for example, on things like telephone mouthpieces).

2. **Swallowing.** Germs that cause hepatitis A and salmonella (food poisoning) ride on human waste and then catch the express on unwashed hands. From there, it's an easy trip to your mouth. (Examples follow.)

Operator's Manual

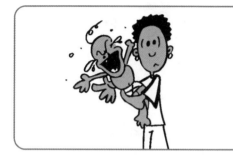

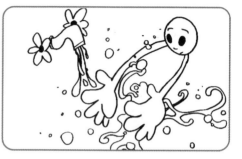

Example A:
A mother changes a baby's diaper, doesn't wash her hands, then prepares a salad.

Example B:
A person goes to the bathroom, doesn't wash his hands, and picks up a slice of pizza.

3. Direct contact. Lice and scabies are passed from one body to another by direct contact. Lice also hitch rides on shared hair brushes and combs.

4. Body fluids. Germs that cause HIV, hepatitis B & C, and STDs travel through blood, semen, and other body fluids.

> ☞ **NOTE**
> The best ways to prevent the spread of disease are to wash your hands, stay out of range when someone is sneezing or coughing, and use a condom during sex.

Sexually Transmitted Diseases

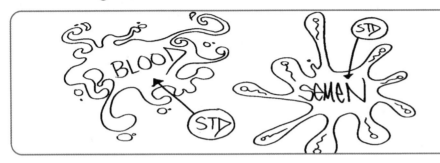

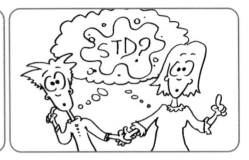

What Are STDs?

Sexually transmitted diseases (STDs) are infections people give or get during unprotected sexual contact (i.e., no condom). The germs travel in fluids: blood, semen or vaginal secretions.

Some STDs have <u>few or no symptoms</u>, so...

- You can spread STDs without knowing it.

- You can't tell if your partner has an STD.

It's important to <u>always</u> use a condom.

Examples of STDs are:

VIRUSES (limited therapy):
- genital herpes
- genital warts
- HIV infection (AIDS)
- hepatitis B*

BACTERIA (can be treated with medication):
- gonorrhea
- syphilis
- chlamydia

*can be prevented with a shot

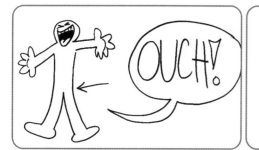

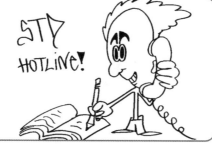

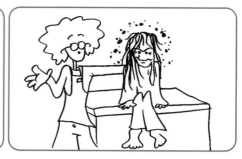

Symptoms of STDs

Go to a clinic or doctor soon if you think you might have an STD or if you have:

- discharge from vagina, penis, rectum
- pain/burning during urination or intercourse
- pain in the abdomen or testicles, buttocks and legs.

☞ **NOTE**
You can call the National STD Hotline:
1-800-227-8922

- open sores, warts, rashes, swelling in the genital area or mouth
- flu-like symptoms: fever, headache, aches, swollen glands.

WARNING!
Don't mess with STDs. See a doctor immediately. STDs can cause permanent damage or, if you are pregnant, can damage or kill your baby.

HIV/AIDS

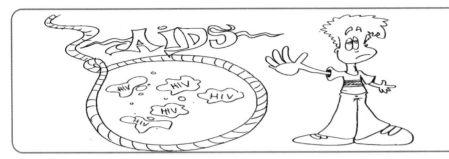 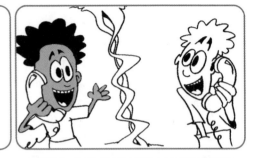

What Is AIDS?

AIDS is an incurable, fatal disease caused by HIV, a virus. Most people who get the virus have <u>no symptoms</u> until months or years later, when they get sick.

People can have and spread HIV long <u>before</u> they have symptoms.

AIDS (**A**cquired **I**mmune **D**eficiency **S**yndrome) breaks down the body's immune system; so people with it get infections that are rare for others to get, especially a kind of pneumonia and a kind of cancer. Their body cannot fight these infections.

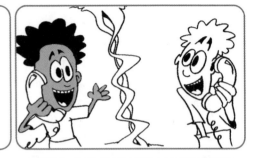
NOTE
You can call the National AIDS Hotline:

1-800-342-AIDS

or the Gay/Lesbian Task Force Crisisline:

1-800-221-7044

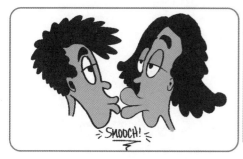

HIV Is Spread Two Ways

1. Sexual/Fluid Contact —
when semen, blood, vaginal secretions (and maybe urine, feces, saliva) enter another's body through the mouth, a cut, an open sore, the vagina or the anus.

2. Sharing Needles —
using IV needles that someone else has used, for drugs, steroid shots, tattoos, piercing, etc.

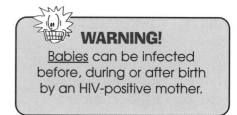

WARNING!
Babies can be infected before, during or after birth by an HIV-positive mother.

The HIV Antibody Test

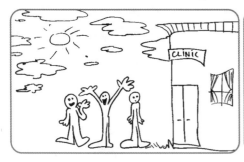 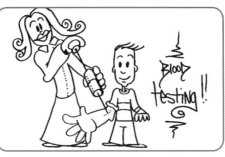 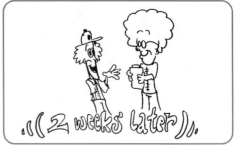

The HIV Antibody Test

The number of people with AIDS is growing rapidly; it is an epidemic.

There is a simple HIV test you can take. A blood sample is taken from your arm. Results come back in 2 weeks. Counselors talk with you both times you go in.

Consider being tested if:

- You have more than one sex partner.

- You've had unprotected sex with a partner whose HIV status you don't know.

- You've had sex with someone who uses needles for drugs.

- You've shared needles.

- A sex partner of yours is HIV-positive.

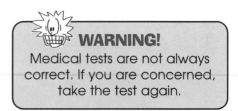

WARNING!
Medical tests are not always correct. If you are concerned, take the test again.

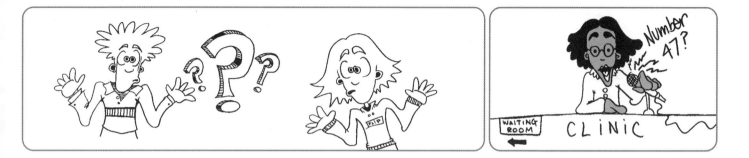

It is important to be tested so you can <u>know</u> whether you are infected.

The test won't work if you got the virus in the last three months, and it doesn't predict the future. You can still get infected anytime.

If you test positive, you may have trouble getting health or life insurance, and you may be discriminated against by your boss or landlord (this is illegal).

☞ NOTE
To avoid possible discrimination by an employer or health insurer, you can go to a clinic that has <u>anonymous</u> testing. You won't have to give your name, address, phone number, or social security number.

Rape

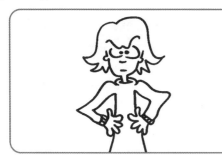
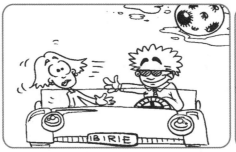
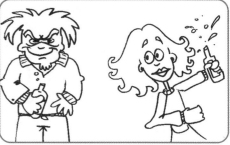

Rape

Being raped, or forced to have sex, has a serious effect on a person's life.

Here are some things you can do to reduce the risk of being raped or coerced:

- Use strong body language.
- Assert what you want and don't want.

- Make good eye contact.
- Use a strong voice.
- Be clear on what your personal boundaries are.
- Pay attention to your feelings and instincts.

☞ **NOTE**

Rape victims need to get checked for HIV and STDs.

⚡ **WARNING!**

FOR TEENS, most of the time (85%), the rapist is someone the victim knows and trusts.

15% of the time, rapists are "strangers" who look for an unsuspecting girl at a party where there is alcohol, then find a way to be alone with her.

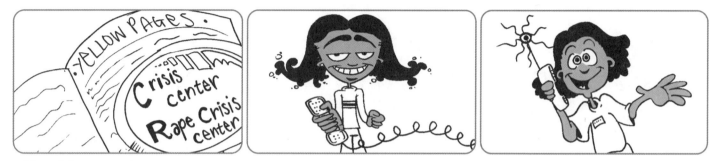

The Aftermath

If you are raped or sexually assaulted, call a rape crisis center right away. You can find it in the Yellow Pages, usually under "Crisis Intervention." People there will help you deal with your feelings, talk to the police, and deal with the courts.

If you are raped, you can choose whether or not to report it. There are legal time limits on filing charges.

In legal cases, it is important to protect as much of the evidence as possible. If you are raped, don't bathe, shower, douche, or wash clothes you are wearing or any materials that were touched such as blankets and sheets until you talk to someone at a crisis center.

WARNING!
An emergency contraceptive pill is available that reduces the chance of pregnancy after intercourse.

Abusive Relationships

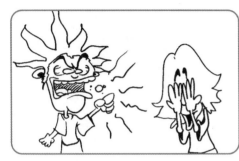
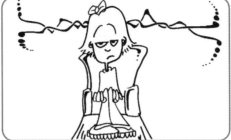
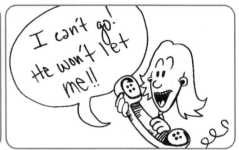

Abusive Relationships

A relationship can turn abusive when one person tries to dominate and control the other person — physically, sexually, emotionally, or financially. Abusive relationships can happen to <u>anyone</u>.

Early Warning Signs of Abuse

Are you going out with someone who...
- is extremely jealous and possessive?
- won't let you have friends?
- constantly checks up on you?
- won't accept breaking up?
- orders you around?
- threatens you?
- is violent?
- pressures you for sex or drugs?
- mistreats you, then blames you for it?
- has a history of bad relationships?

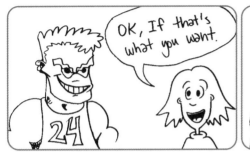 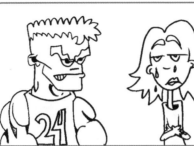 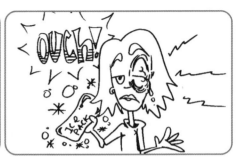

The Vicious Cycle

The abuse in a relationship may not happen right away, but when it does, it goes into a familiar pattern.

At first, everything is really great. Then tension builds. Finally, the tension turns into abuse. Then the cycle starts all over again.

Breaking the Cycle

It may be hard to recognize and break the cycle. If you suspect you are in an abusive relationship, you need help. Find someone with whom you can talk that will really <u>listen</u> and <u>believe</u> you. Look up domestic violence under "Social Service Organizations" in the Yellow Pages.

> ☞ **NOTE**
> One in every four teen girls will be involved in an abusive relationship.
>
> Males can also be victims of abuse.

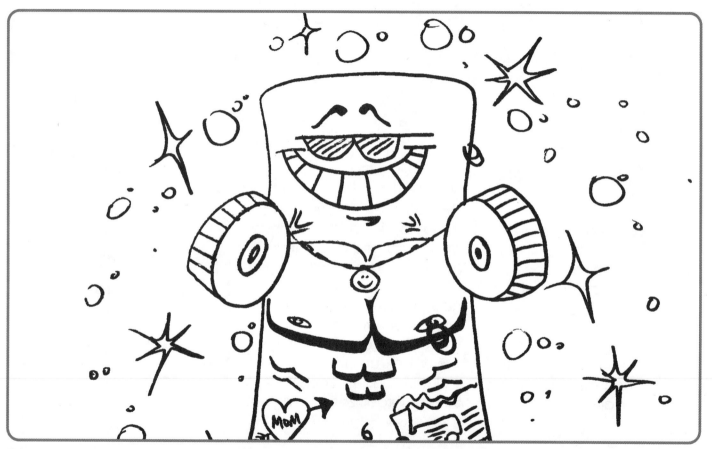

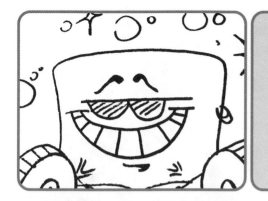

This section has information about customizing the look of your body and the risks involved.

Anabolic Steriods

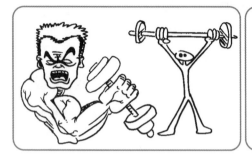

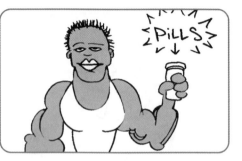

The teen body is shaped by genes, but it also can be remodeled by the owner through exercise, eating, and grooming.

Here are other ways teens customize their bodies — and the possible damages.

Anabolic Steroids

Steroids are a fast way for getting a more buff look or for strengthening the body.

Problems from steroids include:

- They are psychologically addicting.

- They cause acne, aggression, body swelling, mood swings, long-term disease, and depression.

- For women, they cause infertility, baldness, body hair growth, shrinking breasts, and deepening of the voice.

- They are illegal.

Operator's Manual

Eating Disorders

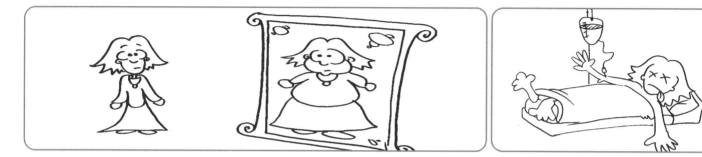

Eating Disorders

Typical eating disorders can include continually eating too little, or too much, or forcing elimination through vomiting or laxatives, or exercising too much.

Eating disorders are most common among teen and young adult females.

Eating disorders can be dangerous and life threatening. If you have any doubt about your eating patterns, talk to a nurse or doctor.

> ☞ **NOTE**
> http://www.anred.com
> is a good website about
> eating disorders.

Are You At Risk?

You may be at risk if you:
- feel "fat" and people say you are thin
- have absent or irregular menstrual periods (girls)
- are secretive about food
- worry about food
- feel guilty about eating
- feel you have to be thin.

People recover from eating disorders, but almost all need help to do it.

Body Art

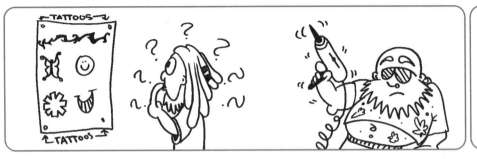 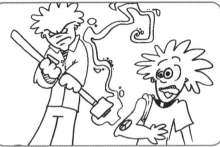

Tattoos

The process of tattooing involves injecting color under the skin. It is relatively painless. About one-third of the time it results in complications, such as infections and diseases. Make sure the practitioner opens a new bottle of ink and a new needle in front of you.

Before getting a tattoo, ask yourself: "How will I feel about this tattoo in thirty years?"

Tattoo Removal

Removing a tattoo is an expensive, time-consuming process that burns and scars the skin.

Branding

Branding involves burning a pattern into skin, which forms a permanent scar. During the process of healing from the burn, the body is at high risk for infection.

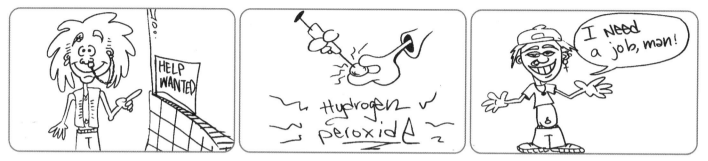

Body Piercing

Body piercing involves poking a hole in the body surface to hold an ornamental object. The process of piercing or the object often causes an infection.

To reduce the risk of infection, be sure:

- all needles used to pierce are sterile
- you use materials that won't cause an infection
- you keep the area free of germs for up to six months with alcohol swabs or hydrogen peroxide.

If infections persist, talk to a nurse or doctor.

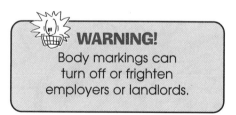

WARNING!
Body markings can turn off or frighten employers or landlords.

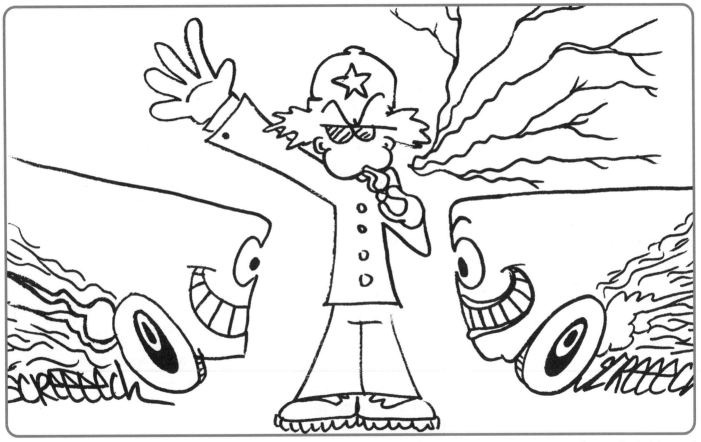

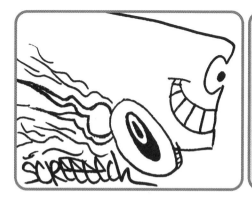

SCREEEECH

Part 7
Sex Brakes

This section gives information about preventing sexually transmitted diseases and unwanted pregnancies.

Safer Sex

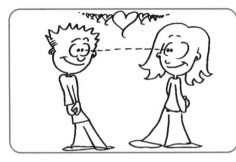

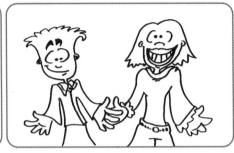

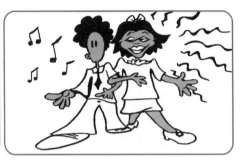

Sex
Your body's reproductive sexual functioning kicks in during pre-teen to teen years.

Safer Sex
"Safer" sex does not mean eliminating sex or pleasure. It means protecting yourself and your partner from STDs or unwanted pregnancy.

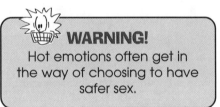

WARNING!
Hot emotions often get in the way of choosing to have safer sex.

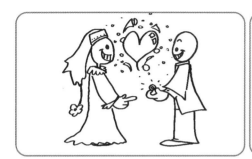 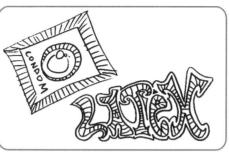 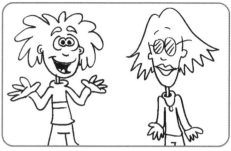

What Works

There are four ways of having safer sex.

1. **Abstinence.** Not having sexual intercourse.

2. **Safe Play.** Talking, fantasizing, touching, massaging, kissing, masturbating.

3. **Monogamy.** Having one committed partner (this still requires using a condom).

4. **Latex Condoms.** When used correctly, <u>latex</u> condoms prevent STDs and pregnancy.

Talk It Over

In a healthy relationship, partners agree on STD protection and birth control <u>before</u> having sex.

Condoms

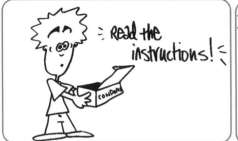

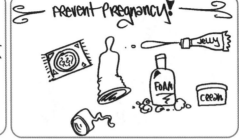

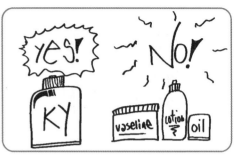

Condoms Prevent STDs

Condoms are an effective way to prevent STDs. Buy latex condoms that say "disease prevention" on the package.

Condoms Prevent Unwanted Pregnancy

To prevent pregnancy, use spermicide nonoxynol-9 (in foams, creams, jellies) — in the tip of the condom and on the outside of the penis, also in the vagina.

If you want lubrication (helps keep condom from breaking) use a water-based variety (e.g., KY jelly), not oil-based (cream, lotion, Vaseline, massage oil).

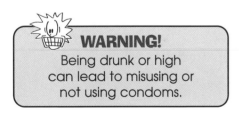

WARNING!
Being drunk or high can lead to misusing or not using condoms.

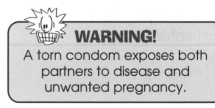

NOTE
There are instructions inside boxes of condoms.
Be sure to read them.

WARNING!
A torn condom exposes both partners to disease and unwanted pregnancy.

Birth Control

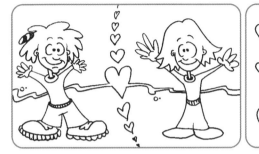

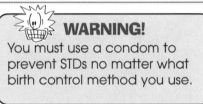

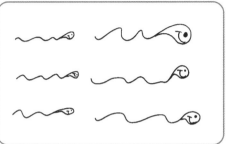

Methods

Pregnancy can happen <u>any</u> time you have sexual intercourse with the opposite sex. If you intend to have sex, use some form of birth control.

There are many methods of birth control:

1. Abstinence

The most reliable method of birth control is abstinence (not having intercourse).

2. Hormonal Methods

a. *The Pill*, for females, contains low doses of progesterone and estrogen. It is prescribed by doctors and taken daily. It can cause lighter periods and fewer cramps.

Birth Control

The Pill is the second most reliable form of birth control.

However, there are side effects, such as moodiness, weight gain, and irregular bleeding.

b. *The Birth Control Shot*, Depo Provera, keeps females from ovulating. It is given every 12 weeks. The side effects are the same as with the Pill. Females may not be able to get pregnant for 1½ years after stopping treatment.

c. *Norplant* is a plastic tube implanted in a female's upper arm, that releases a constant dose of the hormone progesterone for 5 years.

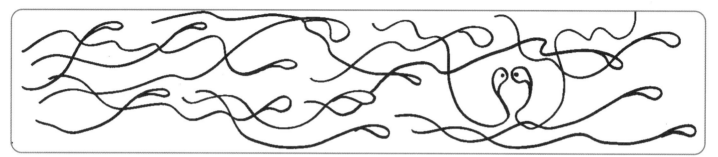

3. Barrier Methods

Barriers for females include: *diaphragm, cervical cap, female condom,* and/or *spermicide.* Barriers for males are *condoms* and *spermicide.*

WARNING!
Using male and female condoms at the same time may cause them to tear.

4. The IUD

The *IUD* (intrauterine device) is a small piece of copper or plastic medicated with progesterone, which is inserted into the uterus. It can cause serious infection, especially if either you or your partner has more than one partner.

5. Sterilization

Sterilization is a surgical procedure — a woman's fallopian tubes are cut and sealed — which <u>permanently</u> prevents pregnancy.

A man can also be sterilized with a *vasectomy.*

Birth Control

More about Vasectomy

Vasectomy is a minor surgical procedure that makes it impossible for a pregnancy to occur, so it is considered permanent.

A vasectomy blocks the tubes that carry sperm from the testicles.

After a vasectomy, sperm continue to be produced, but they are absorbed into the body instead of being ejaculated in the semen when a man "comes" during sexual excitement.

Reversing a vasectomy involves intricate microsurgery and costs several thousand dollars.

Success in restoring fertility is uncertain and cannot be guaranteed. 50-70 percent of men with reversed vasectomies are able to father children afterwards.

Before having a vasectomy, be absolutely certain that you won't want any more children.

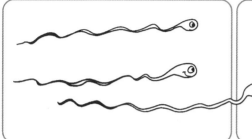

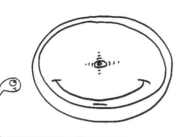

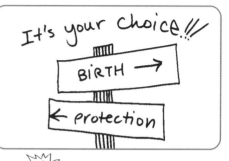

6. Natural Family Planning

It is possible for females to track when they are fertile, but relying on this method is very risky for avoiding pregnancy.

7. Withdrawal

Withdrawing the penis before ejaculating does not work to avoid pregnancy.

Tiny drops near the tip of the penis before ejaculation contain sperm which can travel up to the egg.

WARNING!

Some people think that urinating or douching (washing the vagina) prevents pregnancy.

In fact, this washes the sperm up into the uterus, making pregnancy even more likely.

Other Sexual Issues

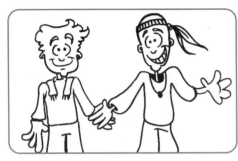 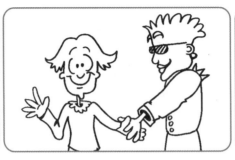 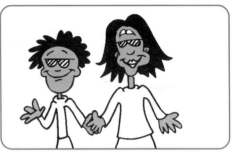

Sexual Preference

Your body-mind gives you messages about your sexual preference as you mature. Sometimes this process is complicated by previous experiences, such as being raped or abused.

Take time to understand your attraction.

Sexual preference has not been an open subject within our culture.

In the past, those who chose a relationship with someone of their own sex often kept it a secret to avoid ridicule and discrimination.

Now society is making a transition toward accepting those individuals into the mainstream, as seen in the media, business, and churches.

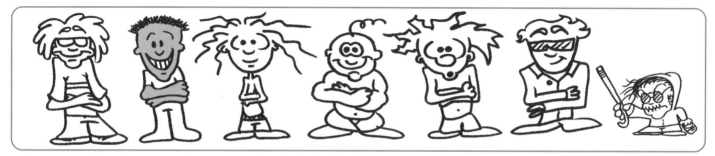

Solo Sex

Often, children touching themselves in the genital area are discouraged by adults, leaving anxieties about this act.

In 1972, the American Medical Association declared masturbation, or solo sex, a normal sexual activity that can ease sexual tension.

According to a study by the Kinsey Institute, 94% of men and 70% of women masturbate.

Safety and privacy are very important when masturbating.

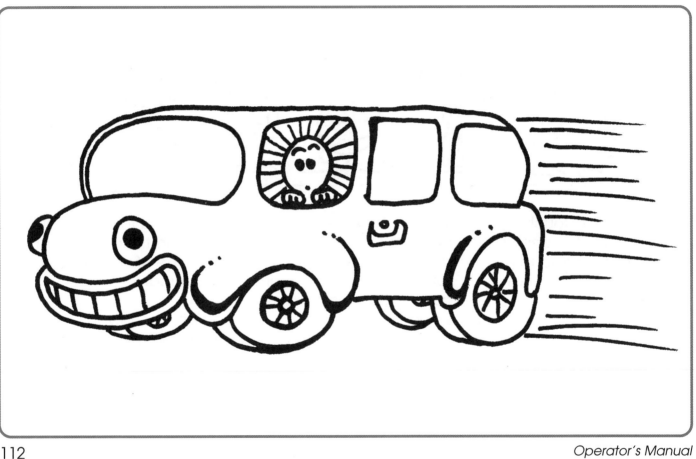

Part 8
Passenger Safety

This section is dedicated to the "passengers" of the human body: unborn babies.

Pregnant?

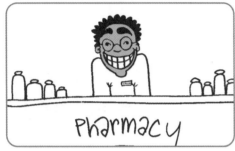

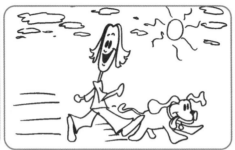

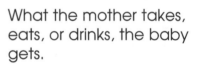

Pregnant?

If you have intercourse and miss a period (especially if you feel very tired or sick), you could be pregnant.

You can get a pregnancy test kit at a drug store. Follow directions carefully. The test works 10 days or more after conception.

The Right Step

If the result is positive, get prenatal care right away, no matter what choice you may make about your situation.

When your body is carrying a passenger, you have to nourish and care for yourself and the passenger.

What the mother takes, eats, or drinks, the baby gets.

Getting prenatal care will guide you in keeping your body and your baby healthy.

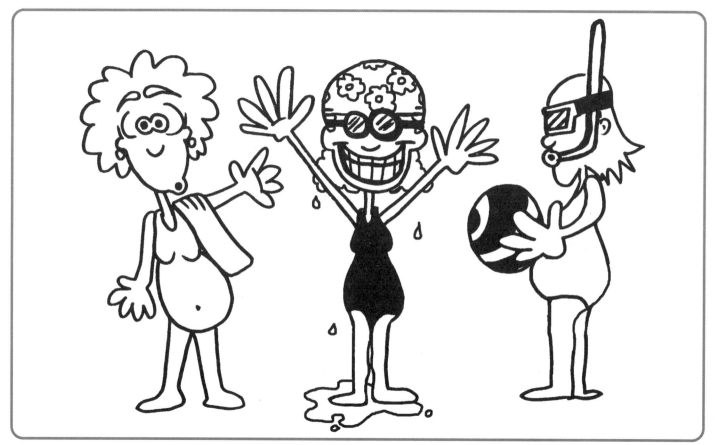

In Harm's Way

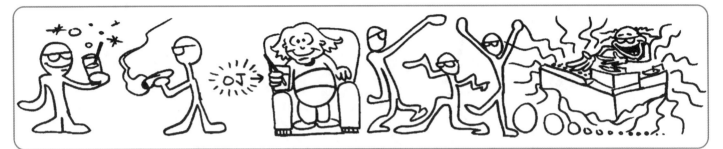

Alcohol
Alcohol reaches the baby quickly, no matter what kind it is. Alcohol can affect the baby's growth, especially the first few weeks of pregnancy, when the baby's body starts to develop.

Women who drink steadily during pregnancy are likely to deliver very small babies who are slower mentally and never catch up.

No one knows a "safe" amount to drink; it's best not to drink at all while pregnant.

Smoking
Babies of women who smoke can be smaller and have more health problems; they can be born too early and have weak lungs.

Caffeine
Cut back or stop eating chocolate and drinking coffee, tea and cola while pregnant. Drink fruit juices or water instead.

Operator's Manual

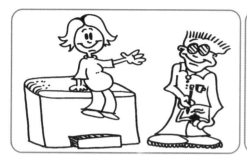

Illegal and Prescribed Drugs

Don't take <u>any</u> medicine, illegal or prescribed, without talking with your doctor.

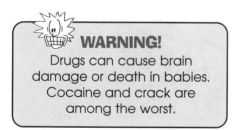

WARNING!

Drugs can cause brain damage or death in babies. Cocaine and crack are among the worst.

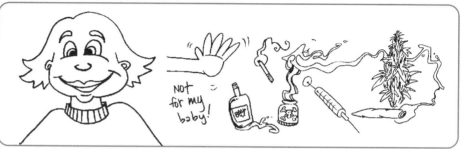

Chemicals

Watch out for the <u>chemicals</u> in your environment, as they can harm your baby.

When you use <u>cleaning products</u>, wear rubber gloves and make sure there's plenty of fresh air where you are working.

Other Dangers

Stay away from <u>paint fumes</u> and <u>insect poison</u> and <u>weed killers</u>.

Don't have <u>x-rays</u> you don't need. Tell the dentist you are pregnant.

Don't sit in a hot <u>hot tub</u>; your baby can't sweat and can overheat!

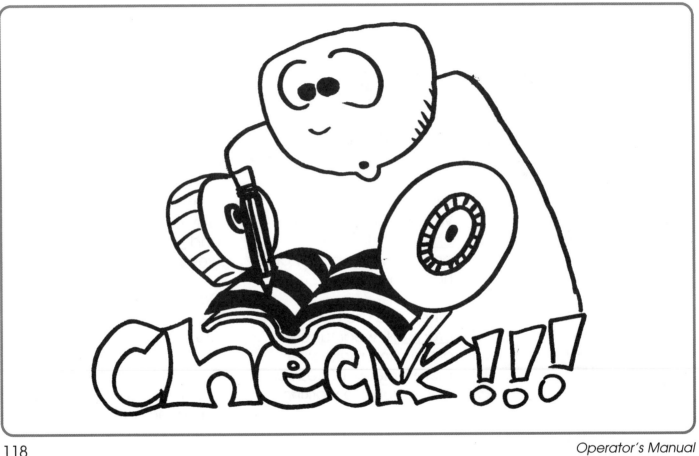

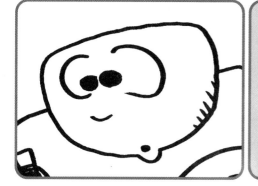

"We are creatures of habit."

Take 20 minutes to look at 99 of your habits.

Instructions:

1. Take out the answer sheet (inside back cover).
2. Go to page 120 and read the first question.
3. Decide which of the five possibilities best describes your behavior in the past six months. Be honest. This is for you alone.
4. Mark one answer — a, b, c, d, or e — on the answer sheet, next to #1.
5. Do the same for the remaining questions.

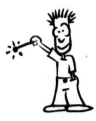

1. I know how to take someone's temperature:
    a. Definitely
    b. Pretty much
    c. Sort of
    d. Not really
    e. I don't know how

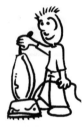

2. I clean my room (wash, dust, vacuum, etc.):
    a. Once a week
    b. Every other week
    c. About once a month
    d. Less than once a month
    e. Never

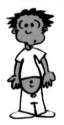

3. When it comes to my weight:
    a. I am within a healthy range
    b. I wonder if I am over- (or under-) weight
    c. I know I should lose (or gain) a few pounds
    d. I am definitely over- (or under-) weight
    e. I have a serious problem

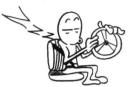

4. I drive when I am tired or ride with drivers who are tired:
a. Never
b. —
c. —
d. I did it once
e. I've done it more than once

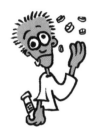

5. I take more than one medication at the same time without knowing how they affect each other:
a. Never
b. —
c. —
d. I did it once
e. I've done it more than once

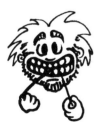

*6. I floss between my teeth:
a. In the morning and at night
b. Once a day
c. Less than once a day
d. Rarely
e. Never

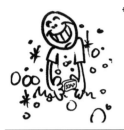

*7. I use soap when I wash my hands:
   a. Every time
   b. Almost every time
   c. Sometimes
   d. Once in a while
   e. Never

8. When I think I'm getting sick, I get medical advice:
   a. Right away
   b. After a day or two
   c. After a week
   d. After more than a week
   e. Never

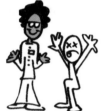

*9. I get enough sleep to feel rested in the morning and alert all day (without caffeine or other stimulants):
   a. All the time
   b. Most of the time
   c. Sometimes
   d. Once in a while
   e. Never

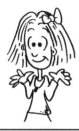

10. When I make a mistake, I still feel OK about myself:
   a. All the time
   b. Most of the time
   c. Sometimes
   d. Once in a while
   e. Never

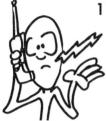

11. I know someone who I can call when I need help or support:
   a. Any time
   b. Most of the time
   c. Sometimes
   d. Not really
   e. No, I don't have anyone like that

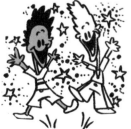

12. I have friends I can trust:
   a. Definitely
   b. Mostly
   c. Pretty much
   d. Not really
   e. No

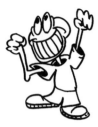

13. I feel good about my accomplishments:
    a. All the time
    b. Most of the time
    c. Sometimes
    d. Once in a while
    e. Never

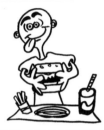

*14. I eat french fries, pizza, hamburgers, hot dogs, fried chicken, etc.:
    a. Never
    b. Once in a while
    c. Sometimes
    d. Most of the time
    e. All the time

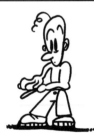

*15. I trim and clean my nails:
    a. All the time
    b. Most of the time
    c. Sometimes
    d. Once in a while
    e. Never

16. I wash and store everything in the kitchen properly:
a. All the time
b. Most of the time
c. Sometimes
d. Once in a while
e. Never

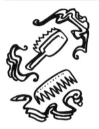

*17. I share my hairbrush or comb:
a. Never
b. Once in a while
c. Sometimes
d. Most of the time
e. All the time

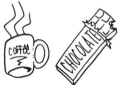

*18. I use products that contain caffeine (coffee, tea, cola, chocolate, and/or pills):
a. Less than once a day
b. About once a day
c. Two or three times a day
d. About four times a day
e. Over four times a day

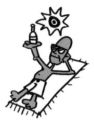

19. I protect myself from sunburn:
    a. All the time
    b. Most of the time
    c. Sometimes
    d. Once in a while
    e. Never

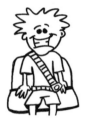

*20. I wear seat belts:
    a. Every time
    b. —
    c. —
    d. I forget occasionally
    e. I often forget

21. If I'm having a hard time (emotionally or physically), I feel OK about getting professional help:
    a. Definitely
    b. Only if it's a crisis
    c. I'm not sure
    d. Probably not
    e. No

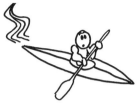

22. Before I take a serious risk, I think and make sure my skills are up for it:

    a. Every time .
    b. —
    c. —
    d. Almost every time
    e. Not usually

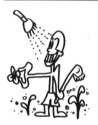

*23. I take a bath or shower:

    a. Every day
    b. Every other day
    c. Every 3 or 4 days
    d. About once a week
    e. Less than once a week

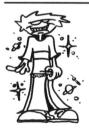

*24. I wear clean and washed clothes:

    a. All the time
    b. Most of the time
    c. Sometimes
    d. Once in a while
    e. Never

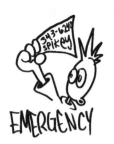

25. I carry with me the name and phone number of someone to be contacted in case of emergency:
   a. All the time
   b. Most of the time
   c. Sometimes
   d. Once in a while
   e. Never

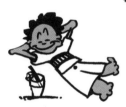

*26. I do things to reduce stress (like relaxing):
   a. All the time
   b. Most of the time
   c. Sometimes
   d. Once in a while
   e. Never

*27. I straighten up my room (put away clothes, shoes, etc.):
   a. Daily
   b. Several times a week
   c. Every week or two
   d. Every three weeks or less
   e. Never

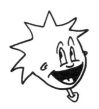

*28. I keep my skin free of dirt, oil, and sweat:
 a. All the time
 b. Most of the time
 c. Sometimes
 d. Once in a while
 e. Never

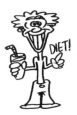

*29. I drink beverages or eat foods with artificial sweeteners (e.g., "diet" soda):
 a. Never
 b. Once in a while
 c. Sometimes
 d. Most of the time
 e. All the time

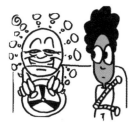

30. I ride with people who are drunk or high:
 a. Never
 b. —
 c. —
 d. I did it once
 e. I've done it more than once

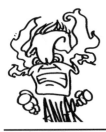

31. I control my anger:
a. All the time
b. Most of the time
c. Less than I would like
d. Sometimes my anger controls me
e. My anger controls me all the time

*32. I can tell people what I want:
a. Always
b. Most of the time
c. Sometimes
d. Once in a while
e. Hardly ever

33. I know how to use First Aid to deal with minor cuts, burns, bumps, and sprains:

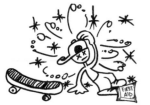

a. Yes
b. —
c. —
d. —
e. No

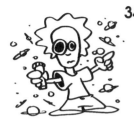

34. I use other people's medications:
a. Never
b. —
c. —
d. I did it once
e. I've done it more than once

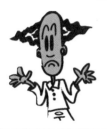

35. I feel hopeless about things:
a. Never
b. Once in a while
c. Sometimes
d. Most of the time
e. All the time

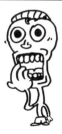

*36. I bite my nails:
a. Never
b. Once in a while
c. Sometimes
d. Most of the time
e. All the time

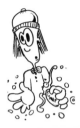

*37. I wash my hands before and after I touch food:
    a. Every time
    b. —
    c. —
    d. Almost every time
    e. Not every time

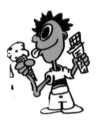

*38. I eat candy, cookies, chocolate, ice cream, etc.:
    a. Never
    b. Once in a while
    c. Sometimes
    d. Most of the time
    e. All the time

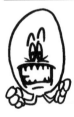

39. I feel stressed:
    a. Never
    b. Once in a while
    c. Sometimes
    d. Most of the time
    e. All the time

40. I drive over the speed limit:

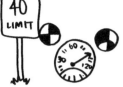

a. Never
b. —
c. This does not apply to me
d. Sometimes
e. Often

*41. I brush my teeth:

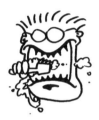

a. Several times a day
b. In the morning and at night
c. Once a day
d. Less than once a day
e. Rarely

*42. I drink water:

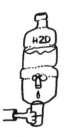

a. About 8 cups a day
b. About 4 cups a day
c. Once a day
d. Almost never
e. Never

43. I know what to do in an emergency situation (how to give CPR, help someone who is choking, or give First Aid):
- a. Definitely
- b. Pretty much
- c. Sort of
- d. Not really
- e. I don't know

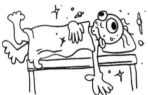

44. I recognize signs of bacterial infection:
- a. Definitely
- b. Pretty well
- c. Sort of
- d. Not really
- e. Not at all

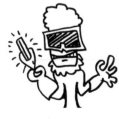

45. I protect my eyes during risky activities (sports, working with chemicals or power tools, etc.):
- a. All the time
- b. Most of the time
- c. Sometimes
- d. Once in a while
- e. Never

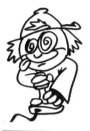

*46. I play video or computer games:
   a. Never
   b. Once in a while
   c. Sometimes
   d. Most of the time
   e. All the time

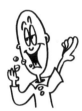

47. I take more medication than the instructions say I should take:
   a. Never
   b. —
   c. —
   d. I did it once
   e. I've done it more than once

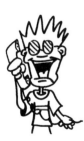

48. When I call or visit a nurse or doctor, I know the details of my symptoms and my medical history:
   a. Completely
   b. Mostly
   c. Somewhat
   d. A little
   e. Very little

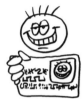

49. I keep my current license, registration, and insurance on me or in my car:
    a. All the time
    b. Most of the time
    c. This does not apply to me
    d. Once in a while
    e. Never

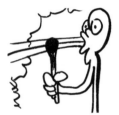

50. I put out matches thoroughly:
    a. All the time
    b. Most of the time
    c. Sometimes
    d. Once in a while
    e. Never

51. I remove health hazards from my house/apartment (e.g., lead paint chips, broken glass, dangerous electrical situations):
    a. All the time
    b. Most of the time
    c. Sometimes
    d. Once in a while
    e. Never

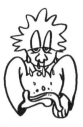

52. I get colds and/or the flu:
a. Very rarely
b. About once or twice a year
c. About once every season
d. About once every month
e. All the time

53. I like myself:
a. All the time
b. Most of the time
c. Sometimes
d. Once in a while
e. Never

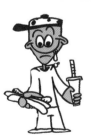

54. I eat a variety of foods, including — bread, cereal, rice, pasta, vegetables, fruits, beans, nuts, milk, yogurt, cheese, meat, poultry, fish, and eggs:
a. All the time
b. Most of the time
c. Sometimes
d. Once in a while
e. Never

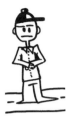

55. I am careful about my personal safety when I'm on the street:
    a. Always
    b. Usually
    c. Sometimes
    d. Rarely
    e. Never

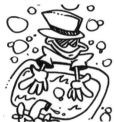

*56. I wash my hands after I use the bathroom:
    a. Every time
    b. —
    c. —
    d. Almost every time
    e. Not every time

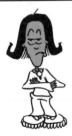

57. I feel lonely:
    a. Never
    b. Once in a while
    c. Sometimes
    d. Most of the time
    e. All the time

Operator's Manual

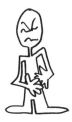

58. I get stomach aches:
    a. Very rarely
    b. A few times a year
    c. About once a month
    d. About once a week
    e. Just about every day

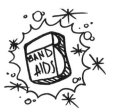

59. In my house, I keep a good supply of First Aid items (Band-Aids, disinfectant, etc.):
    a. Always
    b. Usually
    c. Sometimes
    d. Rarely
    e. Never

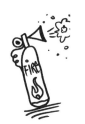

60. Wherever I'm living, I know where to find baking soda and/or a fire extinguisher:
    a. All the time
    b. Most of the time
    c. Sometimes
    d. Once in a while
    e. Never

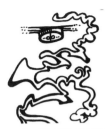

61. When it comes to the smoke alarms in my house:
    a. I check them
    b. —
    c. —
    d. I don't know if they work
    e. I don't know if there are smoke alarms

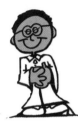

62. I feel happy and satisfied with my life:
    a. All the time
    b. Most of the time
    c. Sometimes
    d. Once in a while
    e. Never

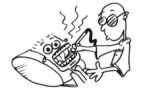

63. I go to the dentist:
    a. Twice a year
    b. Once a year
    c. Once every other year
    d. Rarely
    e. Never

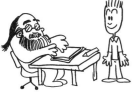

*64. I use good manners when I'm with people:
  a. Always
  b. Most of the time
  c. Sometimes
  d. Once in a while
  e. Hardly ever

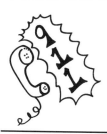

65. I know when it's important to call 911:
  a. Definitely
  b. Pretty much
  c. Sort of
  d. Not really
  e. I don't know

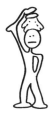

66. I get headaches:
  a. Very rarely
  b. A few times a year
  c. About once a month
  d. About once a week
  e. Just about every day

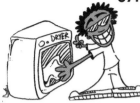

67. I wash and change my bedding and towels:
    a. Once a week
    b. About once every two weeks
    c. About once every month
    d. Less than once a month
    e. Never

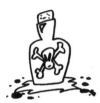

68. I keep poisons labeled and out of children's reach (chemical cleaners, medications, etc.):
    a. All the time
    b. Most of the time
    c. Sometimes
    d. Once in a while
    e. Never

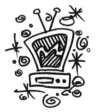

*69. I watch TV:
    a. Rarely
    b. Once or twice a week
    c. About an hour a day
    d. 2 - 4 hours a day
    e. Over 4 hours a day

Operator's Manual

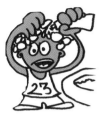

*70. I wash my hair:
a. Every day
b. Every other day
c. Every 3 or 4 days
d. About once a week
e. Less than once a week

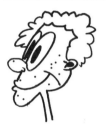

*71. I pick or squeeze my pimples:
a. Never
b. Once in a while
c. Sometimes
d. Most of the time
e. All the time

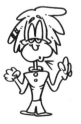

*72. I remind myself to take full breaths (or do an activity that requires full breaths):
a. Many times a day
b. About once a day
c. A few times a week
d. I never think about it
e. I have problems with breathing

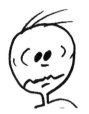

73. I can tell the difference between just having the blues and being really depressed:
  a. Definitely
  b. Pretty sure
  c. Maybe
  d. Probably not
  e. No

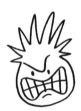

74. I feel like hurting someone, something, or myself:
  a. Never
  b. Once in a while
  c. Sometimes
  d. Most of the time
  e. All the time

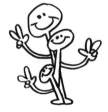

75. I have friends that trust me:
  a. Definitely
  b. Probably
  c. I guess
  d. Not really
  e. No

76. I keep emergency equipment (First Aid kit, spare tire, blanket, etc.) **in my car:**

 a. Yes
 b. —
 c. This does not apply to me
 d. —
 e. No

---

77. Wherever I'm sleeping, I know the exit route to escape a fire:

 a. All the time
 b. Most of the time
 c. Sometimes
 d. Once in a while
 e. Never

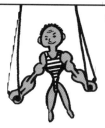

*78. I exercise (or am physically active):

 a. At least three times a week
 b. Once or twice a week
 c. Less than once a week
 d. Less than once a month
 e. Rarely

79. I carry identification and emergency medical information (allergies, special needs) in my wallet:

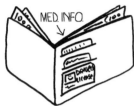

a. All the time
b. Most of the time
c. Sometimes
d. Once in a while
e. Never

*80. I get up about the same time:

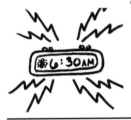

a. Every day
b. Almost every day
c. Sometimes
d. Once in a while
e. Rarely

*81. I drink sodas (pop):

a. Less than once a week
b. Once or twice a week
c. Once a day
d. Two or three times a day
e. More than three times a day

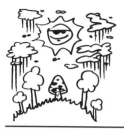

*82. I spend at least an hour a day outside:
   a. Every day
   b. Almost every day
   c. Once in a while
   d. Almost never
   e. Never

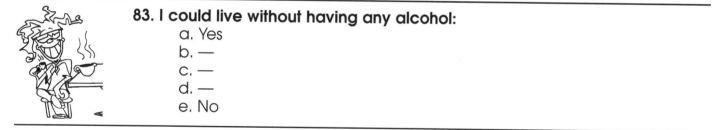

SILENT SURVEY
You may feel more comfortable just thinking about your answers to the following items, rather than writing them down.

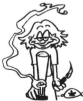

83. I could live without having any alcohol:
   a. Yes
   b. —
   c. —
   d. —
   e. No

---

84. I use illegal drugs (pot, coke, meth, etc.):
   a. No
   b. —
   c. —
   d. -
   e. Yes

85. (If pregnant or breastfeeding) I drink alcohol, smoke, and/or do drugs:
a. No
b. —
c. This does not apply to me
d. —
e. Yes

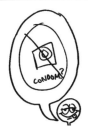

86. I have sex without using a latex condom:
a. No
b. —
c. This does not apply to me
d. —
e. Yes

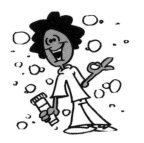

87. I use prescription drugs (tranquilizers, sedatives, uppers) for pleasure:
a. No
b. —
c. —
d. —
e. Yes

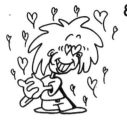

88. I have sex while I'm drunk or high:
a. No
b. —
c. This does not apply to me
d. —
e. Yes

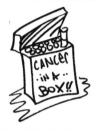

89. I smoke cigarettes:
a. Never
b. Once in a while
c. Sometimes
d. Most of the time
e. Always

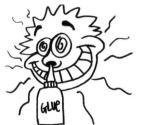

90. I use legal drugs to get high (cough syrup, glue, etc.):
a. No
b. —
c. —
d. —
e. Yes

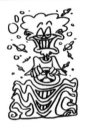

91. I've missed classes or work because of alcohol or drugs (headaches, loss of motivation, etc.);
  a. No
  b. —
  c. This does not apply to me
  d. —
  e. Yes

92. I drive while I'm drunk or high:
  a. Never
  b. —
  c. This does not apply to me
  d. I did it once
  e. I've done it more than once

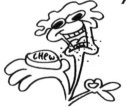

93. I use smokeless tobacco:
  a. No
  b. —
  c. —
  d. —
  e. Yes

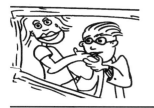

94. I use a reliable method of birth control every time I have intercourse:
a. Yes
b. —
c. This does not apply to me
d. —
e. No

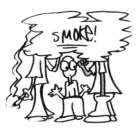

95. I have thought about killing myself:
a. Never
b. Once
c. Rarely
d. Sometimes
e. Often

96. I hang out in places where people are smoking:
a. Never
b. Once in a while
c. Sometimes
d. Most of the time
e. All the time

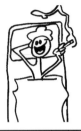

97. I smoke in bed:
a. Never
b. —
c. This does not apply to me
d. Once in a while
e. Regularly

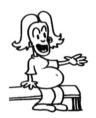

98. I will get prenatal care within the first two months of my pregnancy:
a. Yes
b. —
c. This does not apply to me
d. —
e. No

99. I drink alcohol enough to get drunk:
a. No
b. —
c. —
d. —
e. Yes

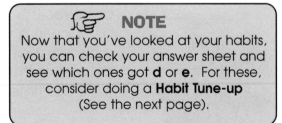

NOTE

Now that you've looked at your habits, you can check your answer sheet and see which ones got **d** or **e**. For these, consider doing a **Habit Tune-up** (See the next page).

Operator's Manual

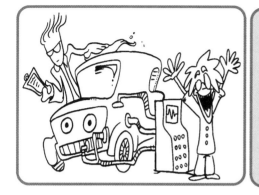

Part 10
Habit Tune-Up

An easy way to improve your health is to change habits that are unhealthy. This section shows a strategy for changing habits.

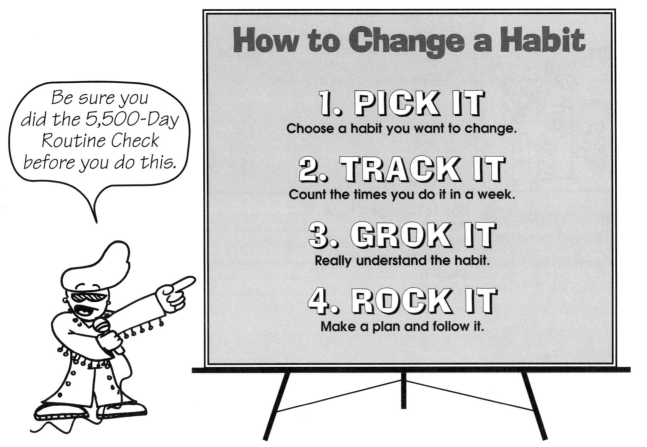

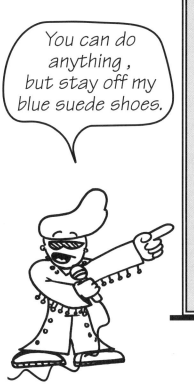

You can do anything, but stay off my blue suede shoes.

1. PICK IT

- Look at the habits listed on pages 157 - 159.

- Choose one of these that you circled ⓓ or ⓔ on your answer sheet.

- Write down the habit you chose on page 160.

- Then, think about why you want to change this habit.

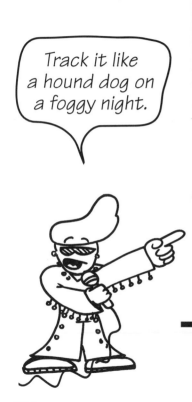

Track it like a hound dog on a foggy night.

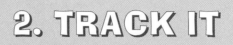

2. TRACK IT

- **Count the number of times you observe the habit.**
(Mark it on a piece of paper, a notebook or your hand.)

- **Enter the daily count on the TRACK IT Summary form on page 160.**

Operator's Manual

Write down every time you:

 6. Floss your teeth

 7. Wash your hands with soap

 9. Feel rested when you wake up

 14. Eat fried or fatty foods

 15. Trim your nails

 17. Share your hairbrush or comb

 18. Eat or drink something with caffeine (coffee, chocolate, soda, diet pills)

 20. Wear seat belts

 23. Take a bath or shower

 24. Wear clean and washed clothes

Continued ⇨

Write down every time you:

 26. Do something to reduce stress

 27. Straighten up your room

 28. Wash your skin gently

 29. Drink or eat something with artificial sweetners

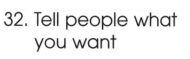 32. Tell people what you want

 36. Bite your nails

 37. Wash your hands before and after touching food

 38. Eat sweets

 41. Brush your teeth

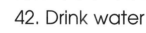 42. Drink water

Operator's Manual

Write down every time you:

 46. Play video or computer games

 56. Wash your hands after using the bathroom

 64. Use good manners

 69. Watch TV

 70. Wash your hair

 71. Pick or squeeze your pimples

 72. Take full breaths

78. Exercise

80. Get up at the same time

81. Drink soda

 82. Spend time outside

 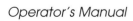

TRACK IT Summary

Habit to track:_____

	Daily Count			
	TRACK IT Week	ROCK IT Week 1	ROCK IT Week 2	ROCK IT Week 3
Day 1				
Day 2				
Day 3				
Day 4				
Day 5				
Day 6				
Day 7				
Weekly Total				

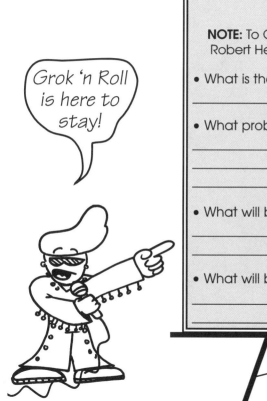

Grok 'n Roll is here to stay!

3. GROK IT

NOTE: To GROK is to understand something thoroughly (from Robert Heinlein's book, **Stranger in a Strange Land**, © 1961).

• What is the habit you are trying to change?

_____

• What problems does the habit create for you?

_____
_____
_____

• What will be the hardest thing about changing the habit?

_____
_____

• What will be the best thing about changing the habit?

_____
_____
_____

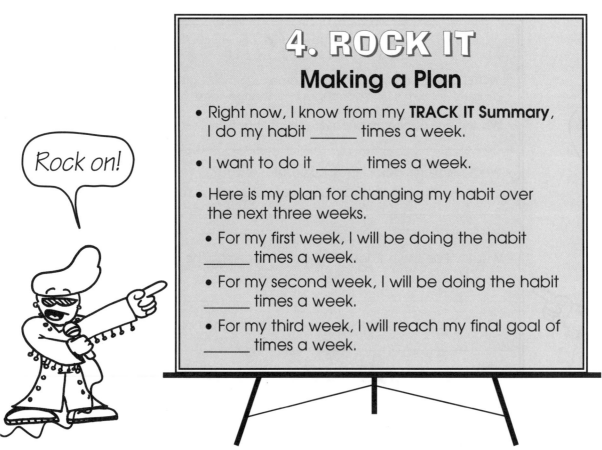

4. ROCK IT
Making a Plan

- Right now, I know from my **TRACK IT Summary**, I do my habit _____ times a week.

- I want to do it _____ times a week.

- Here is my plan for changing my habit over the next three weeks.

  - For my first week, I will be doing the habit _____ times a week.

  - For my second week, I will be doing the habit _____ times a week.

  - For my third week, I will reach my final goal of _____ times a week.

Rock on!

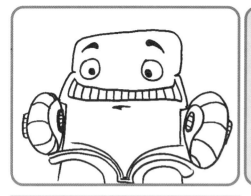

Have a healthy home, starting with these items.

Health-Related Stuff to Have Around

First Aid Supplies

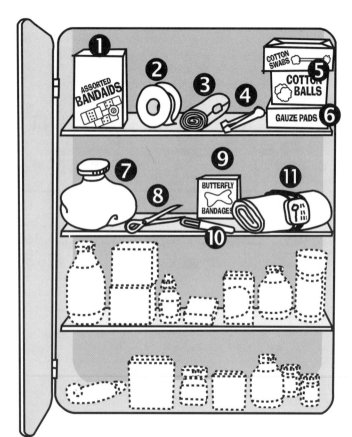

You can put together a First Aid kit by gathering the items listed here, or you can purchase First Aid kits at drugstores or through organizations such as the American Red Cross. Keep a **First Aid** manual (also available at these locations) with your First Aid supplies.

1 **Assorted Band-Aids** — Cover and protect scrapes and cuts from dirt.

2 **Adhesive Tape** — Holds gauze pads in place.

3 **Ace (Elastic) Bandage** — Wraps around sprains and supports injured area.

4 **Tweezers** — Remove dirt and splinters from wounds.

5 **Cotton Balls and Swabs** — Clean out wounds or scrapes.

6 **Gauze Pads** — Cover large wounds or scrapes.

7 **Ice Bag** — Reduces swelling from injuries.

8 **Sharp Scissors** — Cut gauze from roll and remove jagged edges of skin.

9 **Butterfly Bandages** — Hold edges of a cut together.

10 **Thermometer** — Determines presence of a fever.

11 **Heating Pad** — Speeds healing after swelling is reduced and may relieve headaches; use on low.

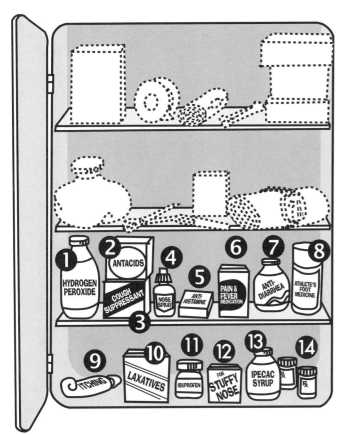

Home Pharmacy

Here are some useful medications to have on hand.
Be careful! (see p. 62, about pills)

1 Antiseptics (Hydrogen Peroxide) — For cleaning wounds and preventing infections.

2 Antacids — For heartburn and upset stomach.

3 Cough Suppressants/Expectorant — For coughing or excess phlegm.

4 Nasal Spray/Nose Drops — For a runny or stuffed up nose.

5 Antihistamines — For a runny nose and itching,watery eyes.

6 Pain/Fever Medications (Acetaminophen, Ibuprofen, Naprosyn) — For pain and fever.

7 Antidiarrheals — For diarrhea.

8 Antifungal Preparations — For fungal infections such as athlete's foot.

9 Skin Irritation Medications (Hydrocortisone) — For itching from bites, poison ivy, etc.

10 Laxatives — For constipation.

11 Anti-Inflammatories (Ibuprofen, Naprosyn - NOT Aspirin) — For swelling and pain in muscles and joints.

12 Decongestants — For a stuffed up nose.

13 Syrup of Ipecac — For poison (induces vomiting). Don't take unless directed to do so.

14 Special Medicines — For personal needs.

Read Up!

*Take Care of Yourself:
The Complete Illustrated
Guide to Self Care
6th ed.
Vickery, D.M. & Fries, J.F.
Reading, MA:
Addison-Wesley
Publishers, 1996

The CareWise Guide:
Self-Care from Head
to Toe
Seattle, WA:
Acamedica Press
(800-755-4400), 1996

Changing Bodies,
Changing Lives
Bell, R., New York:
Random House, 1980

Complete Book of Pregnancy
and Childbirth Rev. ed.
Kitzinger, S. New York: Alfred A. Knopf, 1996

*Responding to
Emergencies: American
Red Cross First Aid
2nd ed., St. Louis, MO:
Mosby Year Book, 1996

The AMA Encyclopedia
of Medicine
Clayman, C., M.D. (Ed.)
New York: Random
House, 1989

How Sex Works
Fenwick, E.& Waller, R.
London, New York:
Dorling Kindersley, 1994

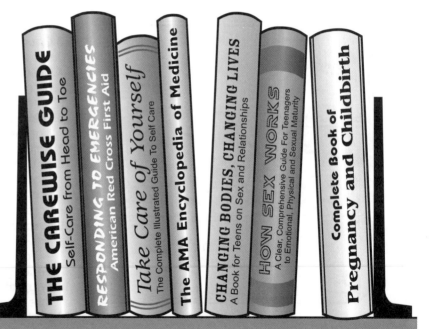

Operator's Manual

Recommended books on health for teens.
The titles with stars are good home
reference books.

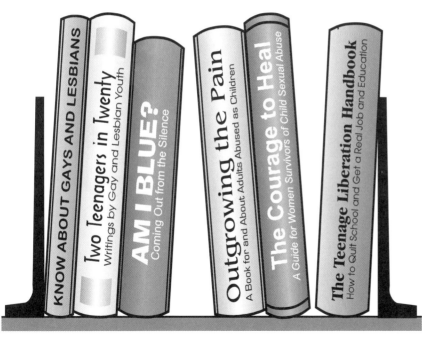

Know About Gays and Lesbians
Hyde, M. & Forsyth, E.
Brookfield, CT:
Millbrook Press, 1994

Am I Blue?
Coming Out from the Silence
Bauer, M., Ed.
New York: Harper
Collins, 1994

The Courage to Heal:
A Guide for Women Survivors of Child Sexual Abuse
3rd ed.
Bass, E.& Davis, L.
New York: Harper
Perennial, 1994

Two Teenagers in Twenty:
Writings by Gay and Lesbian Youth
Heron, A., Ed.
Boston, MA: Alyson
Publications, 1994

Outgrowing the Pain:
A Book for and About Adults Abused as Children
Gil, E., San Francisco,
CA: Launch Press,
1983

The Teenage Liberation Handbook
Rev. ed.
Llewellyn, G.
Rockport, MA:
Element, 1997

INDEX

Operator's Manual

C

Caffeine 80, 122, 125, 157
    addiction 80
    during pregnancy 116
    withdrawal 80
Calcium 26, 29
Calculated risks 74, 127
Cancer, skin 28
Car
    emergency equipment 145
    insurance 136
    license 136
    registration 136
    safety 126
Car accidents 72, 76
Cardiovascular system 13
Cat litter 48
    dangers 36
Cavities 22, 37
Cells 9, 14
Cervical cap 107
Change
    self 41
Chemicals 142
    during pregnancy 117
    reactions 28
    working with 32

Chest pain 54
Chewing tobacco 81, 150
Chickenpox
    spread of 82
Childbirth 167
Chlamydia 84
Chocolate 80, 125, 157
Choking 53, 54, 134
Cigarettes 81, 149
    and fire safety 49
    during pregnancy 116
    quitting 81
Cleaners 142
    household 48
Cleanliness 34-39, 120, 127, 157
Clothes
    appropriate 46
    clean 39, 127
    wrinkled 39
Cocaine 117, 147
Coffee 30, 80, 125, 157
    during pregnancy 116
Colds 58, 137, 165
    spread of 82
Color, seeing 17
Common Problems 58-62

Communication 46
    aggressive 45
    assertive 45, 130
    direct 45
    passive 45
    passive-aggressive 45
Computers 135, 158
Concentration
    loss of 69
Condoms 103-104, 107, 148
    latex 103-104, 148
    prevent STDs 84
    to prevent disease 83
    using 104
Confusion 42
Conjunctivitis (pink eye) 58
Constipation 165
Cooling System 28
Coordination 19
Cosmetics 35
Cough 52, 58, 165
    spreads germs 82
Cough syrup 149
Counseling 42, 65, 126
    for depression 68
Counselor
    finding and choosing 42

Operator's Manual

Operator's Manual

Operator's Manual

5,500-Day Routine Check
ANSWER SHEET
page 1 of 2
Circle one answer per question.

1. a b c d e	*14. a b c d e	*27. a b c d e	40. a b c d e
2. a b c d e	*15. a b c d e	*28. a b c d e	*41. a b c d e
3. a b c d e	16. a b c d e	*29. a b c d e	*42. a b c d e
4. a b c d e	*17. a b c d e	30. a b c d e	43. a b c d e
5. a b c d e	*18. a b c d e	31. a b c d e	44. a b c d e
*6. a b c d e	19. a b c d e	*32. a b c d e	45. a b c d e
*7. a b c d e	*20. a b c d e	33. a b c d e	*46. a b c d e
8. a b c d e	21. a b c d e	34. a b c d e	47. a b c d e
*9. a b c d e	22. a b c d e	35. a b c d e	48. a b c d e
10. a b c d e	*23. a b c d e	*36. a b c d e	49. a b c d e
11. a b c d e	*24. a b c d e	*37. a b c d e	50. a b c d e
12. a b c d e	25. a b c d e	*38. a b c d e	51. a b c d e
13. a b c d e	*26. a b c d e	39. a b c d e	52. a b c d e

53. a b c d e	65. a b c d e	77. a b c d e	88. a b c d e
54. a b c d e	66. a b c d e	*78. a b c d e	89. a b c d e
55. a b c d e	67. a b c d e	79. a b c d e	90. a b c d e
*56. a b c d e	68. a b c d e	*80. a b c d e	91. a b c d e
57. a b c d e	*69. a b c d e	*81. a b c d e	92. a b c d e
58. a b c d e	*70. a b c d e	*82. a b c d e	93. a b c d e
59. a b c d e	*71. a b c d e	Silent Survey:	94. a b c d e
60. a b c d e	*72. a b c d e	83. a b c d e	95. a b c d e
61. a b c d e	73. a b c d e	84. a b c d e	96. a b c d e
62. a b c d e	74. a b c d e	85. a b c d e	97. a b c d e
63. a b c d e	75. a b c d e	86. a b c d e	98. a b c d e
*64. a b c d e	76. a b c d e	87. a b c d e	99. a b c d e